LIFELONG FITNESS 2004

Dr. Bob Delmonteque N.D.

America's #1 Senior Fitness Expert

with Dr. Tony Quinn

www.BobDelmonteque.com
drbobdelmonteque@sbcglobal.net
phone (818) 340-0707

Copyright © 2004 Bob Delmonteque
Longevity Publications

Library of Congress Cataloging-In-Publication Data

Delmonteque, Bob.
Lifelong Fitness 2004 by Bob Delmonteque
ISBN 0-446-39488-2

Front cover, inside front, inside rear cover photos © Melvin Sokolsky
Exercise and gym photos by Robert Reiff and Chris Lund
Nutrition photo by Paula Crane
Posing photos by Bill Dobbins and Woody of Hollywood
Graphic design by Ken Justice
Printed at F.B. Productions, Inc. Chatsworth CA

To everyone who helped me along the way

I would like to offer my sincere thanks to the following people for their generosity, friendship and support over the years:

Joe Weider – Founder of Weider Nutrition and Fitness for his tireless support and encouragement over the last 65 years.

Ray Wilson – My long time training partner and founder of over 500 health clubs around the world, for allowing me the opportunity to help millions of people over a 50 year period find a better way of health.

Bill Hubner – President of Fitness USA for being my best Public Relations man for over 45 years.

Don Wildman – Former President of Bally's Health Clubs for helping me reach new plateaus in aerobic conditioning.

Dick Minns – My old time partner and training partner for spicing up my life.

Ray "Thunder" Stern – President of Stern Air for his friendship and support and helping us reach the impossible dream.

Frank Zane – Owner of Zane Haven and three time Mr. Olympia for fine tuning my body.

Bill Peal – former Mr. Universe for his body building knowledge and support for over 40 years.

Robert Kennedy – Publisher of Muscle Mag International for his constant support for over 30 years.

Denise Du Berry – President of Thane International for believing in me and the youth cocktail system.

Acknowledgements

Dr. Gary Young – President of Young Living for exposing me to a new plateau of essential oil and natural living.

Mark Mastrov – President of 24 Hour Fitness, for giving me the opportunity to work out in his 24 Hour Fitness clubs throughout the world.

David Pecker – President of Muscle & Fitness and American Media for keeping my photo and name in the pubic eye.

Madeline Delmonteque – My wife, partner and coach for helping me for 55 years.

Armond Taney – Senior Editor of Muscle & Fitness and Mr. USA for his help and inspiration in making this book possible.

Glenn Breaswell – For helping me educate millions of people through the Medical Journal of Longevity.

Larry Gurney – President of Rush Health, my grandson, with his youth and blazing determination he helps keep the passion and energy burning inside of me.

Anthony McDonald – President of Hormone R.X., and also my grandson, for continuously keeping me up to date with current scientific information and medical breakthroughs.

Sal Aria – President I.S.S.A. for letting me work with him, helping thousands of people reach for their dreams.

Dr. Robert Young – President of Interlight, for helping me reach my ideal my Ph balance.

CONTENTS

Years ago, when I published a magazine called Your Physique — which later became Muscle & Fitness — the health and fitness industry was relegated to back-alley sweatshops with cast-iron weights. Bodybuilders, weight lifters, professional athletes, and a few Hollywood celebrities were the only ones who took seriously the health benefits of exercise and weight training. Today scientists and other experts are discovering that a life-style dedicated to fitness and good nutritional habits can all but guarantee a longer, healthier life.

For the average person, advancing age means loss of energy, stamina, endurance, and strength. New studies suggest, however, that the changes traditionally associated with aging — increased body fat, reduced bone mass, loss of agility, weak muscles are the result of inactivity as we grow older. But exercise and strength training can benefit adults of any age, and may even reverse the aging process and reduce the risk of certain diseases.

Bob Delmonteque and I have been friends since our youth. We have grown older together and, along the way, have learned a great many things about health and fitness in general, and about aging in particular. Bob is the perfect example of how an active life-style can maximize your shot at longevity and help keep you youthful and strong. At 80 he is in better shape than most men half his age. His golden skin tone and notably chiseled frame have graced the covers and pages of my magazines since the 1940s. In the eyes of many, he is the premier senior model in this country today, and one of my most valuable associate editors.

The training techniques and life-style changes suggested in this book are the perfect solutions to many of the problems confronting an aging society. Bob Delmonteque keeps your mind, body, and spirit buzzing by incorporating the latest in sports technology and nutritional counseling. This book is an inspiring example of Bob's belief that you can be at what you were at 30 — with the proper exercise and nutrition programs.

With mounting medical evidence against the inactive life-style, I recommend *Lifelong Fitness 2004* to anyone who wants to feel and look younger, and live a better quality of life. It's clear that exercise is not limited to the young and spry. Men and women in their thirties and older respond just as well to strenuous muscle training and exercise as younger people. And the numerous benefits — improved strength, increased muscle size, greater freedom of movement — all add up to great muscle reserves in times of stress.

With the right blend of calisthenics, strength training, aerobic conditioning, stretching, sound nutritional practices and certain life-style changes, we all can keep our bodies strong, lean, healthy, and resistant to disease. Even a moderate increase of physical activity can contribute dramatic gains in life expectancy and a sense of well-being. You're never too old. And nothing holds as much promise for a long, healthy, and happy life as a consistent exercise program — especially one designed by Bob Delmonteque.

—Joe Weider, Chairman of the Board,
    Weider Health and Fitness

Here's what world famous anti-aging physicians are saying about Dr. Bob Delmonteque:

Dr. Robert Goldman –

Dr. Bob Delmonteque is one of our prominent longevity icons and a real inspiration. For thousands of doctors in out A4M organization, Bob is a living idol.

> Dr. Robert Goldman
> Chairman A4M Academy of Anti-Aging
> Chicago, IL

Dr. Ron Klatz –

Over the age of 80 Dr. Bob Delmonteque gives us all hope. He is the poster boy of the anti aging movement. Not a doctor alive within the A4M Academy of Anti Aging Medicine doesn't aspire to be like Dr. Bob when he grows up. As for the female doctors, they just all want a date.

> Dr. Ron Klatz, M.D., D.L.
> President A4M Academy of Anti Aging
> Chicago, IL

Dr. Edmund Chein –

Dr. Bob Delmonteque is a prime example of how good you can look and feel in your 80s. Dr. Bob has been a real inspiration to myself and over 5000 anti-aging patients for over 10 years.

> Dr. Edmund Chein, M.D.
> Palm Springs, CA

Dr. Leroy Perry –

Dr. Bob Delmonteque is one of my mentors. His career has been a real inspiration to me and millions of others in the field of health, nutrition and longevity. Dr. Bob has been coming to my office every week for over 3o years to get his adjustment to maintain good posture and good health.

> Dr. Leroy Perry
> President & Chairman Intl. Sports Medicine Institute
> West Los Angeles, CA

Dr. Ron Lawrence –

Dr. Bob Delmonteque is the perfect role model and gives hope to tens of millions of people who want to live life to the fullest. I believe that anyone in their 60s, 70s, 80s, even 90s can get back into shape. Anything in life is possible if you wan it bad enough.

> Dr. Ron Lawrence
> Malibu, CA

Dr. Fouad Ghaly –

I have known Dr. Bob Delmonteque for almost a decade and find him an inspiration not only for myself but for all those who want to enjoy life to the fullest. Dr. Bob is our living legend because he walks the talk. The advice given in this book is nothing less than pure gold. It is the sum total of all the wisdom that keeps him going strong for over 80 years. We are lucky to be privy to this magic.

> Dr. Fouad Ghaly, M.D.
> Torrance, CA

Dr. Brad Frederick –

Dr. Bob Delmonteque has learned to capture the moment fully in this book. He reveals the secret of living life better and better every day in every way. If you're looking for information and inspiration to living a long and abundant life, Dr. Bob's book has it all.

> Dr. Bradley W. Fredrick
> Director, International Sports Medicine Institute
> West Los Angeles, CA

Dr. Robert Braun –

Dr. Bob grows younger as he grows older through his incredible lifestyle. Dr, Bob is a real inspiration to all us anti-aging. In the next decade, I believe we shall see many people in their 70s, 80s even 90s looking like they are only 40 or 50 years old.

> Dr. Robert Braun, M.D.
> West Hills, CA

Dr. Marc Gordon M.D. –

Leading us in the quest for longevity is Dr. Bob Delmonteque who epitomizes the virtue of a well rounded lifestyle. In his 80s, Dr. Bob functions on a level of a man nearly half his age, this is fostered by his unique daily workout, dietary program and supplementation. Following his program will definitely increase the quality of your life, if not the quantity.

> Dr. Marc Gordon, M.D.
> Medical Director Millenium Group
> Medical Director C.B.S. Studios

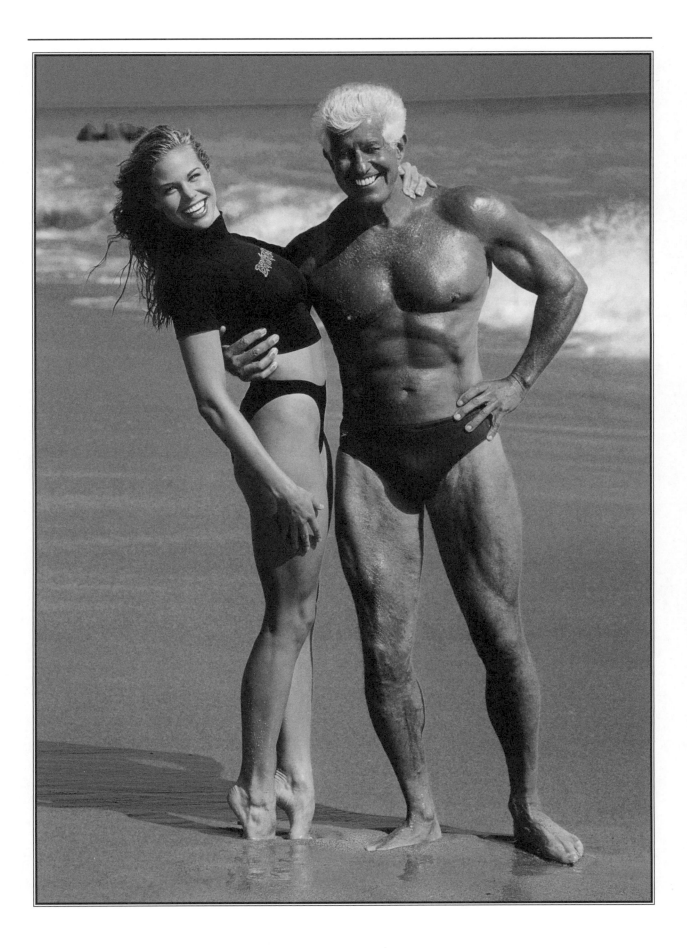

INTRODUCTION

It has been over ten years since I wrote my book LIFELONG FITNESS. It certainly helped raise public awareness to the rapidly sinking state of health of our great nation. It was a huge success and rose above politics and economics in striking at the very roots of our existence, our well being.

So many incredible things have happened to me this past decade I felt I must tell everyone. I'll start right off with the most compelling revelation I've ever experienced, the secret to tapping into my mind, shown to me by the venerable Dr. Tony Quinn. Through my mind I have elevated myself to a new dimension in life: I am actually growing younger in my 80's as I am growing older.

Dr. Quinn and I will bring these nuances to you along with the latest cutting-edge secrets in nutrition, exercise and hormones. I shall also give you my own new daily program, published here for the first time. I believe we can show you how to live to 100 and enjoy every day.

I feel like a man on a mission, one that includes every person on this planet. On my first meeting with Dr. Quinn, I told him that when I was 65 years of age, I felt I was going downhill and began to consider what I could do about it. Would it be possible to defy aging? After some thinking, it finally came to me - I must grow younger as I grew older. My mind made the decision, but it went deeper: My heart sealed it. That was it.

I began to realize that to grow old was a decision, and by making the decision to grow younger I was pioneering an approach everyone could use. I now have the secrets I will reveal to all of you.

When I was exposed to Tony's system, which I believe is one of the best kept secrets in our world, I realized I was already using much of what Tony was teaching. For example, when I made my decision with both my mind and my heart, a passion arose in me to pioneer the way for others. I became so immersed in the dynamics of it that it came to be what I understand to be a program. In short, I think my unconscious mind photographed my unique goal.

This is the secret, the vital foundation. Now my mind, body and spirit are at my all time best. This energy and passion stems from a self-induced experience. I envisioned a bright, white ball of light above me radiating beams of light which I mentally directed to my solar plexus. From there, like something electric, I let the white light radiate throughout my body filling every single cell with energy and passion as never before.

In this program you totally relax deeper than ever before through meditation. We call this energizing. All stress, worries, tensions, fears, problems, phobias - in short, any mental effort that has been tying up the life force in your body has been negated.

I have meditated most of my life. This is the first time I have experienced the freeing up of my own energy. It was like being reborn. Every cell in my body was cleared and activated. What a tremendous feeling came over me, and how energized I felt! In those moments I was able to draw out my life and my life style from within.

I believe that all great athletes and great people do this to some degree. You experience energy and life force like never before. This is unquestionably my greatest rejuvenation and health secret if you desire to stop and reverse the aging process. It is possible for the first time ever to take control of aging, and indeed, health at the cellular level. This approach truly excites me. I'm convinced it is the secret if you are really serious about taking control of your health and your aging process.

You must learn to train your mind. From Dr. Quinn you learn to relax to the point where you can enter the light. I was able to run the white light through the organs, glands and cells in my body. Working together with Tony we designed a program for healing, health, mental positivism, body sculpturing and anti aging. We recorded all of it on audio tape.

As your personal trainer it would take a little time and training to reach the necessary levels. However, based on a lifetime of experience in these areas, if you chose only one, it has to be the mental training to the level of cellular mastery. This is the future. But for the ultimate, ageless and successful way of life, my advice is to use all of these tools.

"Health is there for the taking or the refusing."

BACKGROUND

These days, even middle-aged and older individuals who were never "serious" athletes are starting to exercise in the hope of staving off the effects of aging. It's only natural that we should want to be healthier and more attractive, and free of the physical burdens and complaints of every-day living. Why else would you have picked up this book? You're starting to show and feel your age, so you want to find the safest and easiest way to slow down the aging process. You want to stay young, healthy, and fit, and you want to do it now. Am I right?

What I'm about to reveal to you are the training principles and life-style philosophy that have kept me youthful and strong well into my "golden years." Even though I am 80 years old, pound for pound and inch for inch I've got more energy and vitality than most people half my

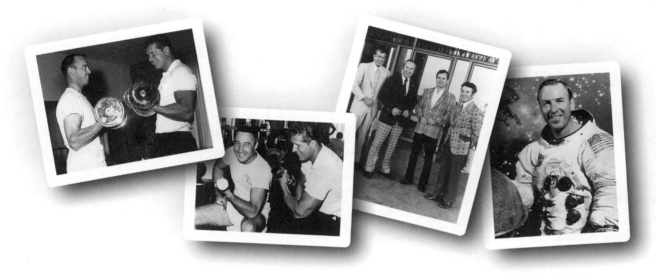

Clockwise from top left: **Bob trains astronaut Alan Shepard; Meeting of the minds: Astronaut James Lovell head of the President's Council on Physical Fitness discussing health and fitness with Bob Delmonteque, Ray Wilson, and Jack LaLanne; Bob with Astronaut Gus Grissom; Captain James Lovell of the Apollo 13.**

age. And that's no brag, just fact. I've traveled from the Far East to the Middle East, from the Scandinavian countries to Mexico, looking for new ways to increase my strength, improve my body, and better my chances at staying young and healthy. I've lived through nearly every gimmick and trend to surface in the health and fitness industry, and I've taken notes on what I've seen and learned.

The truth is your age really has no bearing on your ability to get in shape or fall out of shape, although your attitude can mean the difference between fat and thin, weak and strong, over

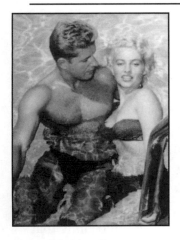

Bob with Marylin Monroe

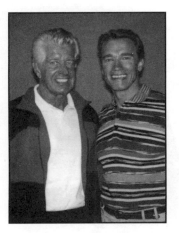

Bob and California Governor Arnold Schwartzenegger

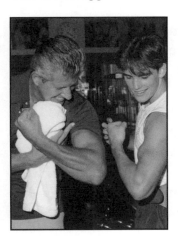

Bob training Matt Dillon

the hill and youthful. When we're young, our bodies are naturally strong, lean, and able to endure the discipline of a demanding life-style. But as we mature, our bodies change in ways we never imagined. Our ability to burn calories diminishes with each passing birthday. Our joints and muscles feel old and tired. Our hearts pump fewer beats per minute. Doctors and scientists have come to recognize what I've known all along — that inactivity makes us more prone to the effects of aging and such illnesses as heart disease, diabetes, and osteoporosis (which affects as many as 24 million Americans, men and women). Preliminary results from a twenty year study at the University of Southern California further indicate that fatigue, weight gain, and even memory loss — often thought to be inevitable as one gets older — may in fact be the avoidable side effects of a sedentary life-style.

Exercise, on the other hand, can give us a better shot at maintaining our strength, stamina, and overall health. It may even prolong youthfulness and reverse the aging process, according to a study at the Human Nutrition Research Center on Aging at Tufts University. The evidence is overwhelming. Even the American Heart Association and the President's Council on Physical Fitness encourage people to exercise as away to enhance well-being and prolong life.

I've trained and reshaped the bodies of personalities ranging from Clark Gable, John Wayne and Errol Flynn to Marilyn Monroe and Matt Dillon. I've counseled some of the nation's best bodybuilders, including Rachel McLish and former three-time Mr. Olympia Frank Zane. Those who have followed my advice have secured contracts with top modeling agencies and won national fitness contests. Others have simply lost that soft spread around the mid-section, thighs, and hips, and reduced the risk of certain diseases. All have discovered the secrets to staying young, healthy, and fit.

Even young people today come to me for advice. They want to know what free-weight exercises I use, what vitamins I take and how they can achieve the energy and vitality that I've achieved. After all, what's the use of living if you can't live life to the fullest of your abilities? My good friend Jack LaLanne once said, "Use it, or lose it." The problem is some people lose it at an early age, while

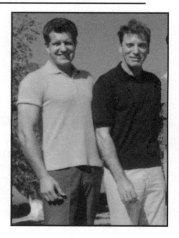

Bob with Burt Lancaster.

others, like me, never stop yearning for new challenges. We hold on to the conviction that we're only as old as we feel. I've got friends in their fifties, sixties, seventies even eighties who water ski and snow ski on weekends, and play golf and tennis on dog days. I've got other friends in their thirties who embrace life with little more than a whimper. What keeps some people rolling in clover fields while others watch the dust settle on their VCRs?

One of the reasons most people have a hard time sticking to an exercise program is that it's often difficult to sift out fact from fiction — from the amount of weight you should be using and the exercises you need to win the battle of the bulge, to your body's special nutritional needs after the age of 30. How much aerobic training is too much? How do you guard against disease and injury?

I don't care if you're 30 years old or 80, man or woman — I'm going to show you how to improve the overall quality of your life. Inside these pages, I'll teach you in one simple, proven program how to build stamina, lose fat and gain muscle and new energy, maintain skin tone and elasticity, brighten your smile, develop rock hard abs, improve your sex life, be as strong and as quick as your younger counter-parts, and slow down and maybe even reverse the aging process. You'll not only live longer, but by your own rules.

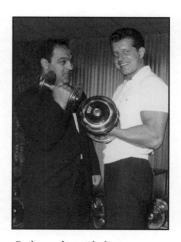

Bob curls with boxer Rocky Marciano

Sound impossible? Well, it's not — and there are no gimmicks, props, or mirrors. I'm the living proof. Most people my age are faced with high blood pressure, heart disease, Alzheimer's, or arthritis — all cruel jokes of Mother Nature. I've never even come close to any of these ailments. I can still run a marathon, bench press 250 pounds, cycle 120 miles, eat and sleep well — and I can show you how to achieve the same results. The Tufts University research taught us that weight lifting combined with stretching and aerobic exercises can help trim body fat, improve flexibility, and make muscles grow stronger in 35-year-olds, 60-year-olds, even 95-year-olds.

But for any program to work you need not only to work your heart, but also to use it. You need to have dreams, faith and goals, pride and self-respect, a blazing determination, persistence, enthusiasm, and, most of all, love for yourself. There's nothing you can't do in life, if you want it bad enough. Nothing!

My training advice and nutritional counseling have had

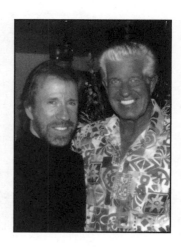

Bob with actor and martial arts superstar Chuck Norris

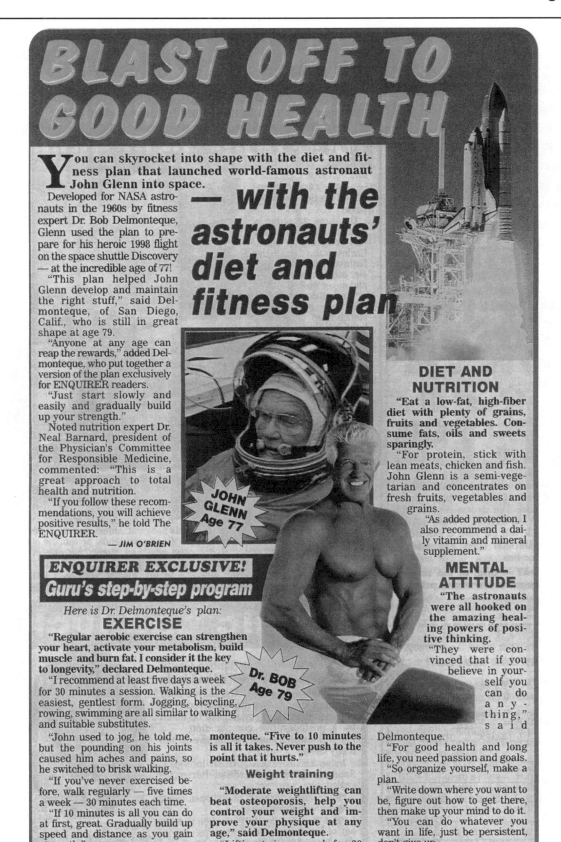

BLAST OFF TO GOOD HEALTH

You can skyrocket into shape with the diet and fitness plan that launched world-famous astronaut John Glenn into space.

Developed for NASA astronauts in the 1960s by fitness expert Dr. Bob Delmonteque, Glenn used the plan to prepare for his heroic 1998 flight on the space shuttle Discovery — at the incredible age of 77!

"This plan helped John Glenn develop and maintain the right stuff," said Delmonteque, of San Diego, Calif., who is still in great shape at age 79.

"Anyone at any age can reap the rewards," added Delmonteque, who put together a version of the plan exclusively for ENQUIRER readers.

"Just start slowly and easily and gradually build up your strength."

Noted nutrition expert Dr. Neal Barnard, president of the Physician's Committee for Responsible Medicine, commented: "This is a great approach to total health and nutrition.

"If you follow these recommendations, you will achieve positive results," he told The ENQUIRER.

— JIM O'BRIEN

— with the astronauts' diet and fitness plan

JOHN GLENN Age 77

Dr. BOB Age 79

ENQUIRER EXCLUSIVE!
Guru's step-by-step program

Here is Dr. Delmonteque's plan:

EXERCISE

"Regular aerobic exercise can strengthen your heart, activate your metabolism, build muscle and burn fat. I consider it the key to longevity," declared Delmonteque.

"I recommend at least five days a week for 30 minutes a session. Walking is the easiest, gentlest form. Jogging, bicycling, rowing, swimming are all similar to walking and suitable substitutes.

"John used to jog, he told me, but the pounding on his joints caused him aches and pains, so he switched to brisk walking.

"If you've never exercised before, walk regularly — five times a week — 30 minutes each time.

"If 10 minutes is all you can do at first, great. Gradually build up speed and distance as you gain strength."

Stretching

"This keeps you limber and prevents injuries," said Delmonteque. "Five to 10 minutes is all it takes. Never push to the point that it hurts."

Weight training

"Moderate weightlifting can beat osteoporosis, help you control your weight and improve your physique at any age," said Delmonteque.

"Lifting twice a week for 20 minutes is enough.

"Start with as little as two to five pounds."

DIET AND NUTRITION

"Eat a low-fat, high-fiber diet with plenty of grains, fruits and vegetables. Consume fats, oils and sweets sparingly.

"For protein, stick with lean meats, chicken and fish. John Glenn is a semi-vegetarian and concentrates on fresh fruits, vegetables and grains.

"As added protection, I also recommend a daily vitamin and mineral supplement."

MENTAL ATTITUDE

"The astronauts were all hooked on the amazing healing powers of positive thinking.

"They were convinced that if you believe in yourself you can do anything," said Delmonteque.

"For good health and long life, you need passion and goals.

"So organize yourself, make a plan.

"Write down where you want to be, figure out how to get there, then make up your mind to do it.

"You can do whatever you want in life, just be persistent, don't give up.

"And laugh, smile, be happy. It will make it easier to follow your dreams."

noticeable results for tens of thousands of people over the past 50 years. My program can be learned quickly and less expensively than any other program on the market — and you don't have to follow a triathlete's training schedule to keep your waistline down and your energy level at full throttle. Anyone — regardless of age, sex, or ability — can benefit from my program, and it's simple and stress-free. With the right mental attitude and a little self-discipline, *Lifelong Fitness 2004* can take you to a whole new dimension of good health and good living.

What You Can Expect from This Program

Here are just a few of the changes you'll notice after only a six-week commitment to my program:

- Stronger and firmer muscles and bones, from a combination of resistance training and weight lifting
- Improved flexibility, mobility, and coordination, from stretching exercises
- More stamina, endurance, and energy, the natural result of aerobic conditioning
- A better shot at losing the right kind of weight, thanks to greater muscle-mass and a higher activity level
- A lower risk of heart disease and high blood pressure, from a low-fat diet and cardiovascular exercise
- A stronger and more efficient heart, the result of a conditioning program that forces your heart to pump more blood with each stroke
- Improved self-image, the result of taking control of your body and your life
- Improved mental abilities, according to a study in 1989 by a psychologist at Scripps College in California
- A better outlook on life because you'll feel better, look better, and develop a more youthful you.

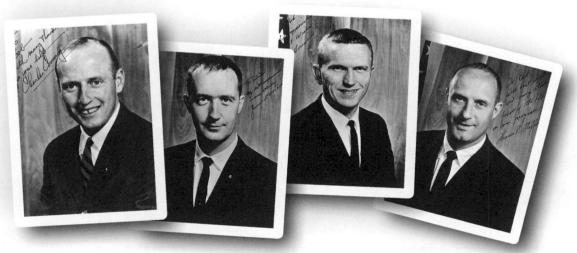

Astronauts Charles Conrad, Jim McDivitt, Frank Borman, Tom Safford

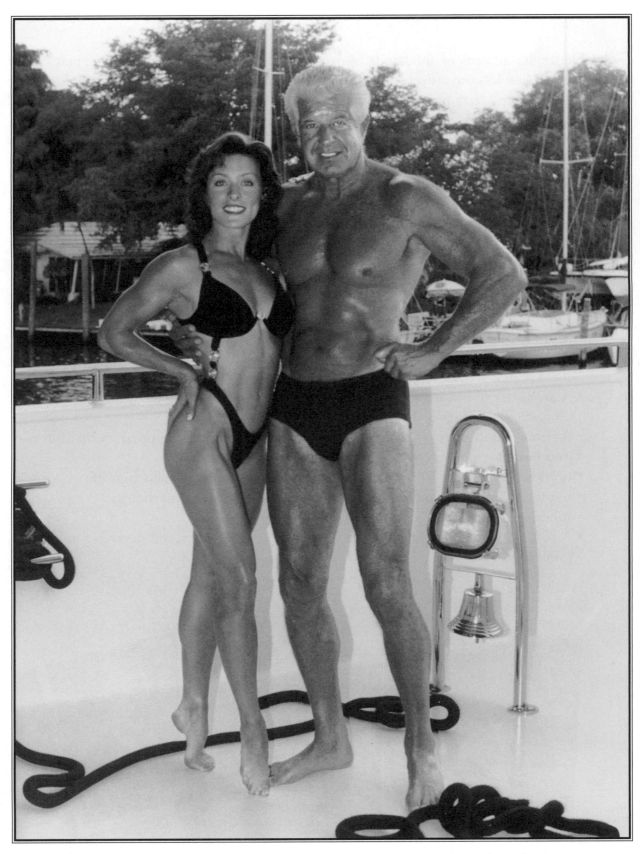

Bob with Kim Peterson

Common Myths about Aging and Fitness

It's amazing how little some people seem to know about the subjects of nutrition, health, and aging. Newcomers to the fitness world are the worst offenders. They not only lack the fundamentals, but they also create their own rules. They drink diet soda with their french fries so they don't feel guilty about the cheeseburger. They play golf-in-a-cart and call it exercise. Sometimes even those who have been exercising for years have erroneous ideas about how their bodies work, especially when confronted with the issue of aging. Ignorance about your health can be the one costly mistake of your life. So before we begin, you must first rethink a lot of what you already think you know.

There's no way on this Earth to turn back the clock of aging.

Some of us age gracefully while others don't, but it has little to do with genetics or anti-aging creams. The average person can lead a longer, healthier, and more productive life by learning a little self-discipline, and by breaking down a few physical and mental barriers. I firmly believe you're only as old or as young as you feel — your chronological age is merely a gimmick for the greeting card industry. Keeping active can push back those barriers, and may even slow down and reverse the signs we typically associate with aging. Lifelong fitness is a viable option — and you don't have to be a professional athlete or eat bran muffins to reap the benefits.

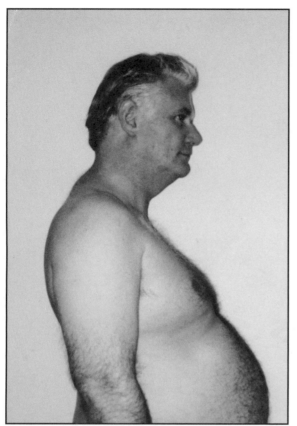
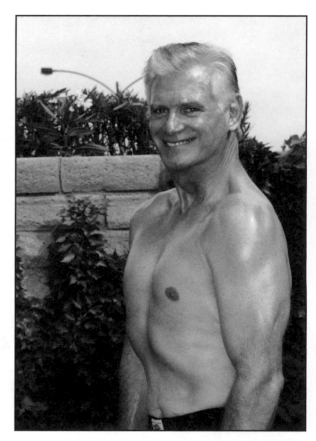
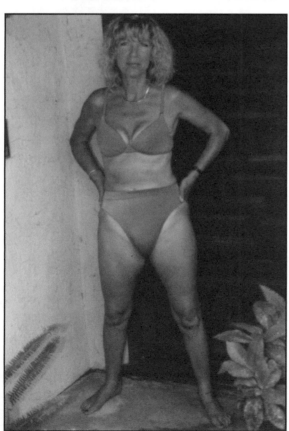
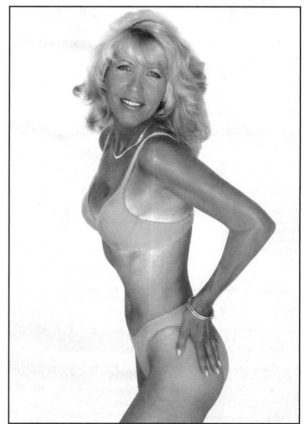

The older we get, the more physical limitations we encounter.

Loss of muscle mass and strength as you get older can mean scaled down mobility and independence. This physical frailty imposes restrictions on everyday activities, and may even trigger injuries. Avoid the ills of inactivity — which result in neck, shoulder, and lower-back pains, headaches, and obesity — and you'll avoid many of the limitations associated with aging. Do whatever it takes to keep active because the more active you become, the fewer physical limitations you'll encounter. All it really takes to keep fit is the determination and the ability to enjoy life. You have choices in life.

Facing Page:

Above: Kevin Knox, age 55, before and after Dr. Bob's program.
Kevin lost 68 pounds and 13 inches off his waist in 5 1/2 months.

"Thanks to bob a whole new life opened up to me. I've actually come out of the closet and started living a new vibrant lifestyle. I was a part time schoolteacher and now I've become a model for commercials and an actor in the movies. this was all achieved under the guidance of Dr. Bob and his program of physical, mental and spiritual. I believe what I have accomplished is possible to anyone who tries."

- Kevin Knox.

Below: Ilsa McMannius, age 60, before and after Dr. Bob's program.
Ilsa lost 32 pounds and 9 inches off the waist in 3 1/2 months.

"It was like the quest for the impossible dream coming true. I recaptured my youth and allure from fashion modeling days. Dr. Bob set me up with an exercise program; and a low carb, low fat, high protein diet.I never accepted the adversity of aging and being over weight, and I believe that Dr. Bob is the reason I regained my youth."

- Ilsa McMannius

Older people can't build muscle and strength like their younger counterparts.

The ability to increase strength, muscle mass, and endurance is not the exclusive privilege of the young. According to the landmark study at Tufts University, exercise can benefit adults of any age and may even reverse some of the signs associated with aging. Additionally, people past middle age can gain muscle and increase strength by as much as 200%. I've seen people in their seventies build muscle, and people in their eighties run marathons. I'm actually in the best shape of my life. I have more muscle mass and density than I've had at any other time because I have a commitment to fitness and have been using the proper techniques to achieve that goal. The only reason I don't lift as much as I did 30 years ago is that we have a tendency as we get older to be more susceptible to injuries, so I've dropped the weight on purpose to reduce my chances.

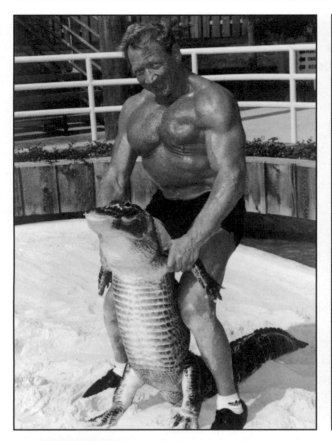

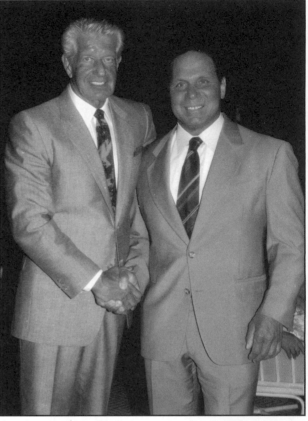

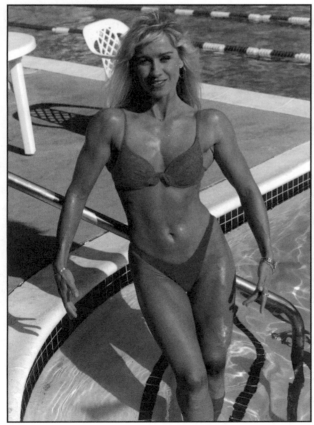

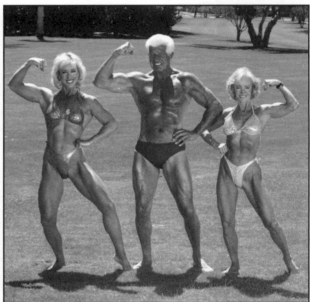

Growing old isn't for sissies: (Clockwise from top left) 70 year old ex-wrestling champion Ray "Thunder" Stern; Bob with 71 year old bodybuilder Bill Pearl; Colleen Fisher age 45, Bob age 80, Kelly Nelson age 75; Lennita Ericson age 40.

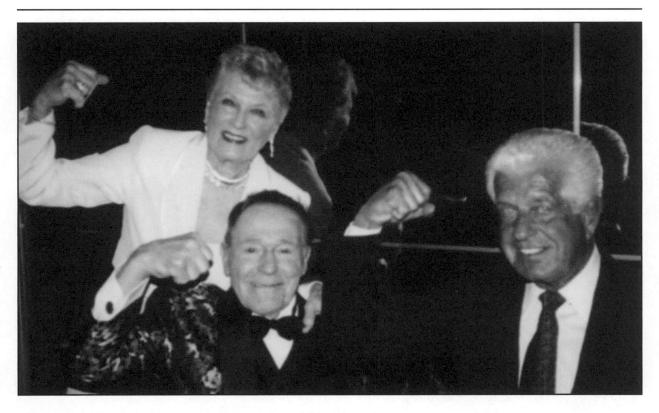

Above: Bob with Elaine and 90 year old Jack LaLanne.

Below: Bob working with President Ferdinand Marcos, helping the Phillipines implement a country wide fitness program.

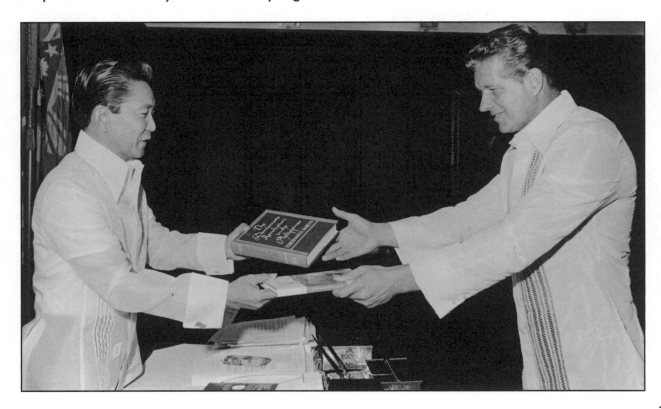

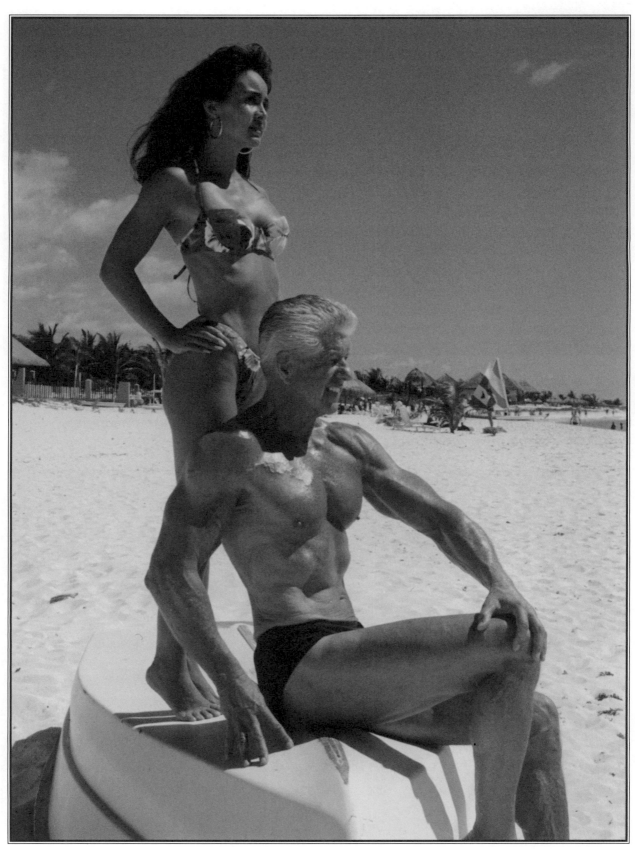

Bob with Miss Mexico Rachel Diaz in Cancun

The body's bone structure eventually becomes too weak to endure the demands of a vigorous workout.

Roughly 24 million older men and women in the United States suffer from osteoporosis (loss of bone mineral and density). The major causes of this decline are lack of physical activity, lack of weight training, and an improper diet. Most people lose about 1 percent of their bone mass per year because as we age we are less able to absorb calcium. The result is weaker bones. Considerable evidence, however, suggests that exercise and weight training delay and may reverse the loss of bone density, especially in post-menopausal women. The added stress that weight training in particular exerts on a bone actually causes it to get stronger, not weaker. Researchers at Tufts University agreed that a consistent weight-training program can, at any age, effectively reduce the rate of bone loss. The solution is to substitute activity for inactivity.

A person over 35 has a harder time burning fat than a younger person.

Anyone, regardless of age, can burn fat. It just may take a little longer if you're over 30 and out of shape. When you last tried to get in shape, did you do too much, too fast? Did you jog around the neighborhood, only to stop in mid-stride with a muscle strain? Did you hop on a stationary bike crank up the tension, and pedal long and hard — only to gasp for air five minutes later? Or did you lift too much weight and damage ligaments? *The basic secret of weight loss is to gradually increase aerobic exercise while reducing saturated fats and complex carbs.*

A slow, steady pace and a realistic program will burn off more fat in the long run than short bursts of exhaustive exercises.

The amount of time you put into your program is more important than the intensity. This program will start you on activities such as light jogging or walking, as opposed to spurts of high-intensity exercises like wind sprints, and you'll train your muscles slowly by lifting the appropriate weight. It takes patience, persistence and discipline but, by increasing your lean muscle tissue, you can continue burning fat at any age. Walking at a brisk pace is about the single best exercise you can do, try to walk 2 miles in under 20 minutes. Motivate yourself and join the 60 million Americans who are out there walking.

Heavy weight lifting causes high blood pressure in older people.

Actually, according to several studies, weight training can help people reduce, and possibly even prevent, high blood pressure. For example, scientists at the Cooper Clinic Institute for Aerobics Research in Dallas reported several years ago that people who keep up with a fitness program stand a better chance of lowering their risk of hypertension. Another study at Northwestern University Medical School in Chicago revealed that resistance training and drinking less alcohol may actually prevent high blood pressure. Normal blood pressure is around 120 over 80, although readings may vary depending on age and other factors. I've been lifting weights since I was 14 years old, and my blood pressure hasn't changed one iota.

People over 35 sustain more injuries than those under 35.

The only times in my life that I ever experienced muscle soreness or injuries were when I either failed to stretch and warm up properly or when I let other concerns interrupt my regular fitness program. Exercise shouldn't cause you injuries or soreness. Naturally, if you're out of shape and attempt the impossible, you're going to feel miserable after an intensive workout. But the main reason people injure themselves is that they use improper form or lift too much weight. In order to avoid injury, stick to my program and follow my instructions concerning proper weight and the intensity of your workout.

Once you're well into your 30s, it becomes hard to improve your cardiovascular system.

Your heart and lungs need a good workout, just like your biceps and triceps. If they are not properly exercised, they will deteriorate with age. As with muscle building, however, aerobic exercise will boost the power of your lungs, your heart, and your body's vascular network. Greater oxygen intake means more oxygen-rich blood that can be carried to the muscles by a stronger cardiovascular system. Strong muscles and a low-fat diet increase your oxygen utilization, which will keep you strong, make you feel and look younger, burn fat, and increase your life expectancy. My doctor says I'm in as good shape as a cross-country skier, which means I can exercise more with less effort. What's my secret? I've work at it, and I let nothing stop me. At the age of 80 I ran a full 26 mile Marathon.

An older trainer needs to work twice as hard as his or her younger counterpart.

Contrary to popular belief, scientists have found that older trainers increase their strength at about the same rate as those who are younger. The now famous results of the Baltimore Longitudinal Study revealed that a healthy older person's heart pumps just about as well as that of his younger counterpart. Naturally, overtraining is a problem, especially for beginners and older trainers. To build and maintain muscle, you should train three times or more per week. If you want to grow stronger, you should increase your weight and intensity gradually over time.

By the time men and women reach 40, they should take life a little easier, make fewer demands on their bodies and muscles, and get more rest.

Study after study suggests that the changes we traditionally associate with aging-weakened muscles, increased body fat, reduced bone mass — are typically the result of inactivity and immobility. In fact, at no time in your life should you retire to the rocking chair on the front porch, even if you're "old" and frail, because once you consign yourself to that chair, you'll never leave it. Naturally, rest is important if you're maintaining a rigorous exercise schedule. It allows your body time to repair itself, to achieve the positive benefits we seek from training (increased muscle mass, improved cardiovascular conditioning). But scientists and doctors have come to realize that extended periods of rest (or inactivity) only make matters worse.

If you want to stay in shape as you age, and stay healthy, you need to stick to a diet.

"Diet" leaves a bad taste in my mouth. It smacks of deprivation and punishment. I urge you to instead think of it as sensible eating habits. What's sensible? Eat everything as close to nature as possible. Stay away from such bugaboos as salt butter, junk food, and refined sugars. Also, cut down on your calories if you're consuming too many, and eat the proper food combinations. Quite simply, if you're overweight you're probably eating too much fatty food and exercising too little. Diets, however, are not the answer. People tend to go on a diet, lose the weight, then gain it back after several months of bad resumed habits. Reducing your daily intake of bread, potatoes, rice, pasta and saturated fats is an excellent beginning.

The ideal way to lose weight is to exercise and to consume the right kinds o of food, those that are low in fat content and calories, and high in flavor. And the benefits of eating this way aren't restricted to weight alone. For example, according to the Fred Hutchinson Cancer Research Center in Seattle, older women reduce their chances of breast cancer by eating less fat, while older men reduce their chances of clogged arteries and heart attacks.

Protein should also be an important part of your diet. I know there are a lot of doctors out there who claim that you need to cut down on your protein intake as you age. They say too much protein causes the body to excrete calcium, which may lead to gout, arthritis, or osteoporosis. But I attribute a good portion of my condition to the fact that I maintain a diet high in protein. Every day I consume a gram of protein for each pound of body weight, or roughly 200 grams of protein daily (mainly of fish and chicken breast). It helps keep my muscles well fed. Of course, I also drink a lot of water to wash away the excess poison in my system. I'll explain more about this concept in Chapter Ten.

No amount of exercise or advice will help me. I'm too far gone.

My program will benefit you in ways even your doctor can't imagine. Everything you need to stay lean and fit and to slow down the aging process is here. If you can still walk, you can do my program. I've learned over the years that the only true way to stave off the effects of aging is to stick to a program that will work. I've tried every trick device, strategy, and concession known to the health and fitness world. I've worked on my body as a mad scientist would, tinkering and trying out experiment after experiment until, finally, I've got it right. Soon it will all come together for you, too: more confidence, better health, mastery over your life, and success in your lifetime battle against the advancing years.

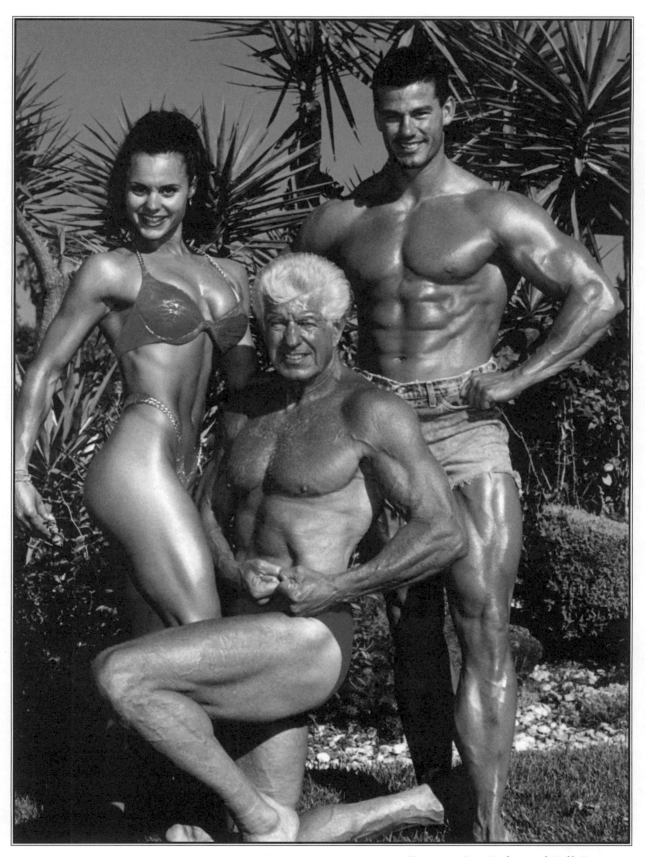

Timea, Dr. Bob and Bill Davies

The Art of Body Maintenance

A person will think of every excuse in the book for why he or she can't exercise: I'm too tired. I don't have the time. I have too many aches and pains. I'm getting too old. Most people believe that exercise is a worthy endeavor, yet many have a hard time sticking to a program. They may feel it's a waste of time for them personally, or that exertion is uncomfortable. Most of all, they may worry that their time would be better spent accomplishing something more productive — as if there's something out there that's more important than one's health. More and more studies are proving that sedentary people don't live as long or enjoy health that's as good as those who get regular exercise. Obesity, especially, has adverse effects on health and longevity, and is a silent contributor to heart disease, high blood pressure, strokes, diabetes, liver and kidney problems, and, as the latest research suggests, perhaps even cancer.

Why suffer when all that can be avoided through simple exercise? The health benefits of exercise are enormous. Weight lifting, for example, may actually reduce the risk of diabetes, according to a study at the University of Maryland. Researchers tracked nine men, ages 50 to 65, for 12 weeks. The men worked out on weight machines for 45 minutes, 3 days a week. Not only did their strength increase, as expected, but so did their insulin sensitivity, which reduces the risk of diabetes. Another study at the Sinai Hospital in Baltimore revealed that resistance training can be useful in the rehabilitation of cardiac patients.

If the studies don't mean anything to you, just look at your peers. While some age gracefully and with few health problems, others, for all practical purposes, look 10 to 15 years older and suffer from more than one ailment. Luck has little to do with it. Those who don't age do things differently from those people who do age. They exercise. Some people claim my genetic code is the only reason I'm not only living longer, but living better. Picking the right parents helps, but few of us get that option. My parents weren't spectacular physical specimens; in my case, I simply realized the enormous mental, spiritual, and physical health benefits of exercise at an early age. I didn't even notice any real physical changes to my body until I reached my sixties. My hair started turning gray, the texture of my skin became more coarse, and my body sagged just below the biceps and around the obliques, or "love handles." But overall I've been in great shape most of my life because 24 hours a day I'm conscious of what my fitness and health goals will yield. But from age 65, I got in the best shape ever, peaking out at age 78.

Now That You're Ready, Where Do You Start?

Naturally, any program of exercise should be approached with caution. The first require-
ment is to see your doctor. Most medical experts suggest that you don't dive head first into an
exercise program. It's best to start slowly. For the sedentary and/or obese elderly person, I recommend the following:

- A medical check up (including a blood panel and stress tests) and your
  physician's OK, with special precautions for persons with cardiovascular
  problems.
- For beginners, a weight or resistance-training workout no longer than
  15 minutes, 3 days a week.
- Five minutes of aerobics (at 60 percent to 75 percent of your maximum heart
  rate), 3 times a week. (Maximum heart rate equals 200 minus your age.)

Set realistic goals. If you want to lose 20 pounds, first set a goal of 5. If you want to walk
two miles, first make it around the block. Don't allow frustration or failure to sidetrack your goals;
remember, if you miss one workout, there's always tomorrow. And give your body a full day's rest
after each workout. It takes time for your muscles to recover.

The first five weeks are the key to your whole future. Once you've established a routine,
you'll be spoiled by the refreshing benefits of the workouts, and your body will demand attention
from you. Let's face it, what you want is to get in shape through very little effort. You want to lose
weight and regain vigor. If you exercise in moderate amounts and make small but intelligent
changes in your eating habits,you can have it all.

The following maintenance program works well for beginners because I've devised a mul-
titude of exercises that anyone can do using common items found in the home. Instead of barbells, I use an ordinary towel. Instead of dumbbells, I use my own opposing strength. It's a great
way to keep your body firmed, toned, and in good shape, without having to buy expensive weight
equipment or commit yourself to a long-term gym membership. Although this program is
designed for people who have never started an exercise program and for those who have long since
given up, it holds benefits for people at any level of fitness — I still train under this program when
I'm traveling and when I get burned out at the gym.

If you're a beginner to the fitness world, it will take you roughly a month before my program kicks in and you begin to notice certain changes, but those with the lowest fitness levels will
also show the fastest improvements. Gains in strength, flexibility, and coordination will come
quickly during the first few months of my program. Those of you who have been training for a
while should use this section to enhance your existing program. Champion bodybuilders often use
a combination of the following stretches and exercises, in conjunction with their regular routine,
to further achieve their fitness goals.

Now that you're ready to begin your exercise program, remember to keep at it. Don't quit at the first sign of frustration. If you're worried about hurting yourself, skip to Chapter Six — Tenets for Preventing Injuries — before proceeding here. But don't let your fears or your natural inertia get in the way of pursuing lifelong fitness. Regardless of your fitness level, learn to tackle your exercise program with your head, your humor, and your heart. And never surrender. There is nothing in life that you cannot accomplish if you want it bad enough.

The following is a simplified version of the program which is laid out in detail further in the book, along with now to breathe properly, more stretches and how-to exercises, and recipes.

EXERCISE

Day 1 - Monday

Chest, Triceps, Shoulders (Stretching after every set of exercise)

Chest
• Bench Press	3 x 10
• Incline Press	3 x 10
• Pec Deck or Dumbbell Flyes	3 x 10

Triceps
• Triceps Extension	3 x 12
• French Curl	3 x 12
• Triceps Kick Back	3 x 12

Shoulders
• Seated Shoulder Press	3 x 10 w/dumbbells
• Upright Row	3 x 12 w/barbells
• Side Lateral	3 x 12 w/dumbbells

Sit-ups
100

Life Cycle
20 minutes

Day 2 - Wednesday

Thigh and Calf

• Leg Extension	3 x 12
• Leg Curl	3 x 12
• Leg Press - Machine	3 x 12
• Standing Calf	3 x 12
• Leg Back Stretch	

Day 3 - Friday

Back

• Lat Machine	3 x 12
• Dumbbell Rowing	3 x 12 Standing - Bent over
• Rowing Machine	3 x 12 Seated

Biceps Curl

• Barbell Curl	3 X 12 Standing
• Dumbbell Curl	3 X 12 Seated
• Dumbbell Concentration Curl	3 X 12 One Arm - Seated

Hints

- • 1. Always maintain good posture when working out.
  Don't lean forward or back, or swing the weight for the sake of momentum.
- • 2. Use my 2 – 4 system
  - – Count of 2 on the way up
  - – Count of 4 on the way down
  - – Positive Up - Negative Down
  - – Muscle is built on the Negative Down side of the sets.
- • 3. Start by using your top weight for 12 reps, then work down.
- • 4. Always maintain good rhythm and form.
- • 5. Exhale when exerting power.
- • 6. Concentrate and visualize the body part you are working. Send messages to that part of the body.
- • 7. Tackle your workout with a great life force. Photograph your goals at a low, unconscious level. (read Dr. Quinn's chapter)
- • 8. Get that surge of energy and passion from within.

Stretch after each group of sets. Change your workout program every three months. Your clever body develops an efficiency over time that tends to slow development.

"As long as a man breathes, he must exercise his body as regularly as he eats his meals if he would maintain top health."

MY DAILY ROUTINE

- I normally awaken about 7 A.M.
- Roll over to my carpet and meditate for 15 minutes.
- I run the Dr. Tony Quinn Program.
- Do my Yoga for 15 minutes which activates my cells. At the cellular level I feel full of vim, vigor and vitality.
- Take my measurements - body weight and waist measurement.
- Shave.
- Massage my face - using a cream and rubbing my face with 100 upward strokes with my palm and massaging around my eyes.
- Brush my hair back with two hog bristle brushes 100 times.
- Floss my teeth and brush with an electric brush.
- Take a hot and cold shower with a massage head.
- Use a 60-inch towel to briskly dry myself until my body is pink.
- Use tear drops to polish the whites of my baby blues.

And I am ready to go.

MY DAILY EATING PROGRAM

Breakfast

- Glass of hot water with lemon juice and apple cider vinegar
- 6 oz. Green Drink
- Fruit - grapefruit or melon or one or two pieces of fruit
- Bran or Irish oat meal w/blueberries
- One or two soft boiled eggs
- One slice of course grain toast if desired
- Green tea or coffee
- Piece of fruit every 2-1/2 hours

Lunch

- Baked potato or yam with piece of fruit in season

                          or

- No fat or low fat cottage cheese or yogurt, or either fish or chicken breast, a piece of fruit

Dinner

- 6-8 oz. fish, chicken (without skin) or a turkey burger or steak (without fat)
- No complex carbohydrates - bread, potatoes, rice, pasta, beans
- Salad w/ Weight Watchers low fat dressing and any veggies:
          broccoli
          cauliflower
          carrots
          mushrooms
          peas
          carrots
- Desert - jello or fruit

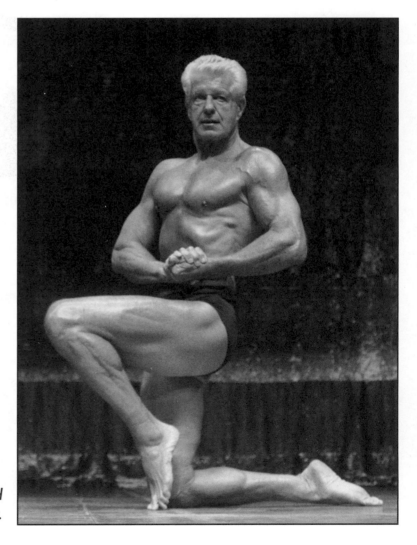

Bob at 72, working the crowd at a bodybuilding show.

Food Supplement

- All around vitamin-mineral
- Anti-oxidants
- Flax seed, black currant oil, wheat germ, soy lecithin pearls

NO-NOs!!!

- 1. No fat - butter, margarine, salad dressing
- 2. No junk food or fast food
- 3. No diet drinks or regular sodas
- 4. No refined sugars
- 5. Minimum dairy products - milk, yogurt, cottage cheese
- 6. No heavy foods at night
- 7. No salt
- 8. No alcohol
- 9. No liquids with meals

GOLDEN RULES

- 1. Eat slowly – chew your food thoroughly and you'll eat half as much
- 2. Drink plenty of water daily
- 3. Eat fruit every 2-1/2 hours
- 4. Complex carb snack only once a day in the afternoon
- 5. Eat 12-16 oz. protein daily
- 6. Eat 3 regular meals with fresh fruit (or nut and seed) snacks every 2-1/2 hours
- 7. Do Swedish Breathing in A.M. and P.M.

In the evening I do 100 sit-ups, take a bath using Dr. Young's Essential Lavender oil, brush my hair 100 times and massage my face. I am ready for bed.

"You may stay young gracefully instead of growing old gracefully by diet and exercise and clean living."

MOTIVATION

God Gives You Choices in Life:

In one hand	*On the other hand*
To be slim	Fat
To be healthy	Unhealthy
To be free of disease	Diseases
To live long	Not to live long
To enjoy life to the fullest	To be miserable

In the end, in order to crystallize the meaning of all I've said, you need motivation. It amounts to a simple decision to live the most extraordinary existence possible.

When you go to bed, you find yourself with an insistent desire to reach the excitement of tomorrow, to find your way back to yourself and to give yourself the gift of a body that can lift and excite you all your life. Body, mind and spirit: The secrets to a healthy body and eternal youth are as simple as eating well, exercising regularly, using your mind and nourishing your soul. Breathe fresh air, keep the faith, and decide to bring bliss into your life. Act, without ever giving up, to bring the bounty of health and well being into your life.

Be patient. So often people give up just before a major breakthrough in fitness or nutrition, typical of their lives in general.

It takes 21 consecutive days of action to change a habit. Anticipate the journey ahead. Begin walking it ever so slowly, and before you know it, you will be running with the energy you used to believe was only for toddlers and teens.

God gives you choices in life, to look good, to feel good, and to enjoy life to the fullest, or you can choose not to look good and feel good and to be miserable and sick. Along with your positive choices, you've got to have goals and dreams, strength and courage and a blazing determination and enthusiasm. But most importantly, you've got to persist until you succeed. You can never give up.

You are what you eat and think. When it comes to living life, you must generate thoughts in a positive direction.

I believe I can do anything I want to do without fear or apprehension. That's the secret to longevity. Don't worry. Be happy. Enjoy yourself to the fullest and help others do the same. Longevity depends on spiritual well being and mental prowess.

NUTRITION

Nutrition is the most important essential to good health. What you eat today you walk and talk tomorrow. Every part of your body is made up of the foods you eat. Try to eat all food as nature provided with no additive and with no preservatives.

Your weight is in direct proportion to the amount of calories you take in a day. It has been determined you need 10 calories per pound of body weight daily:

My body weight - 195x10=1950, my daily, basic calorie intake.

It takes 3200 extra calories to put on one pound. If you are eating more calories than you are expending, you shall gain weight.

OBESITY

Obesity is the #1 killer. You never read about it in the obituary column, but obesity is the killer that hides behind many of the diseases of our civilization:

- Heart, liver and kidney diseases
- High blood pressure and stroke
- Diabetes
- Cancer

HORMONES

Hormones as a key to aging intervention have also been the subject of experiments in aging of the biological clock. Menopause and andropause are the direct results of the fall in sexual hormones HGH, testosterone and estrogen. The organs and glands of the body stop performing at optimal levels. Your body then starts losing lean muscle tissue, becomes wrinkled and flabby and puts on ugly fat. Your hair starts to turn gray and begins falling out, your joints become stiff, you get aches and pains, your energy and sex level diminish, and you have started to age.

I believe this problem could have been prevented with hormone control and a lifestyle of exercise, proper nutrition, mind control and spiritual development. You must fine tune your hormones:

- 1. H.G.H.
- 2. Testosterone
- 3. Estrogen
- 4. D.H.E.A.
- 5. Thyroid

After age 40 most people experience a hormone decline. Your doctor can determine this by arranging a hormone blood panel test to show your hormone deficiencies and prescribe for you:

Testosterone:

- Effects your libido
- Increases sex drive
- Increases aggression which dissipates your depression
- Increases physical strength
- Builds anti bodies and a better immune system

Estrogen:
- Increases vitality, energy
- Reverses thinning of skin and drying of mucous membranes
- Prevents osteoporosis, arteriosclerosis
- Decrease in heart attacks and strokes

H.G.H.
- Lean muscle mass
- Thicker skin
- Look years younger
- Get your sex back
- Lose fat and gain muscle
- Get back your youth

Thyroid
- Regulate metabolic rate of the body
- Prevent cognitive impairment
- Can lower cholesterol levels
- Mental alertness
- Prevent lethargy
- Helps control your weight

D.H.E.A.
- Has been dubbed the mother of hormones
- Protects against arteriosclerosis
- Improves cardiac function
- Lowers blood pressure
- Increases immune factors
- May prevent fat accumulation

I believe hormone therapy along with a proper lifestyle is the wave of the future. In the next two or three decades you shall see 80-year-olds looking like they are 50 coming out of the doctors' offices. Many will be living beyond 100 and still enjoying life to the fullest.

Stem Cells

Researchers the world over are trying to unlock the potential of stem cells in treating a number of ailments. The expected power to do this is astounding. Meanwhile, the stem cell 'immortality gene' has been found. The key gene that keeps embryonic stem cells in a state of youthful immortality has been discovered. It holds the power to treat damaged or diseased organs. Until now scientists did not know how a stem cell renews itself or develops into a new kind of cell. It appears to be the "master gene" that coordinates other genes to allow stem cells to multiply limitlessly while still retaining their ability to differentiate. This immortality gene has been named "Nanog" after the land in a Celtic myth whose inhabitants remain forever young.

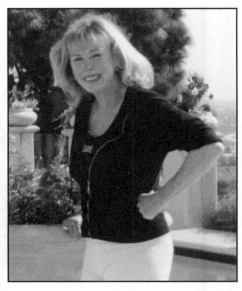

Sonja: fit, happy and well.

Sonja Wilson, at age 58, was diagnosed as having the fifth stage of breast cancer, and her doctor gave her 6 months to live. By luck I knew Dr. James Mason at M.D. Anderson Cancer Hospital in Houston who was conducting an experiment in stem cell therapy. He told me of a program at Memorial Sloan-Kettering Cancer Center that could possibly help Sonja.

Sonja went into the program – first they gave her kemotherapy for several months, then they started the stem cell program. While in the hospital, the doctors drew out 200 million white blood cells along with some of her bone marrow, cleansed the cells and froze them, leaving her with just red blood cells. She was put into an isolation room for 30 days to prevent the risk of infection – then they replaced her clean white blood cells along with stem cells and bone marrow. Within the week, she was discharged from the hospital – and six weeks later she was hiking in the swiss alps.

Today, 8 years later, she is in perfect shape and following my program. God gave Sonja a miracle.

"Health is always unfinished business."

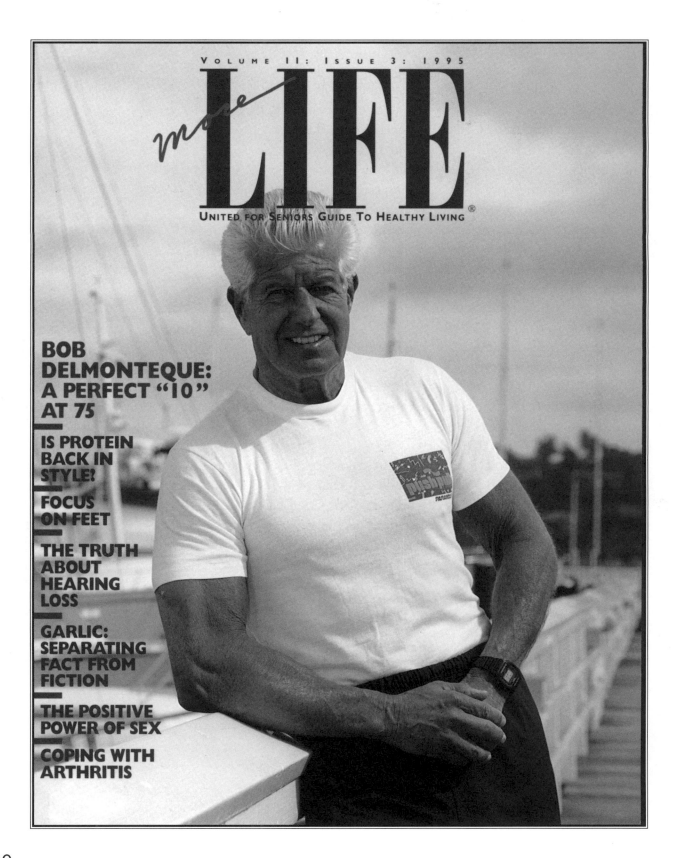

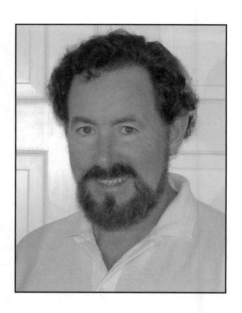

Tony Quinn holds a Master of Science degree in Psychotherapy and Mind Programming, a Doctorate in Counselling and Clinical Hypnotherapy. Presently he is in the process of completing a PhD in Psychology based on the Educo™ System.

Dr. Tony Quinn and the EDUCO™ System

Tapping in to your Subconscious Power

I have never believed in reinventing the wheel. Therefore, when I found the person who was the best in a particular field, the starting point in my research was, to pick their brain. One of my qualifications is in Behavioral Modeling. Behavioral Modeling enables one to draw out the pattern of behavior that made the person exceptional and then make it available to those who wish to achieve similar results.

Over many years I had seen pictures of Bob Delmonteque in health, fitness and body building magazines. Always, I was struck by the inner glow of health that seemed to light up this man and made him stand out in any crowd. Often his picture would appear with some of my

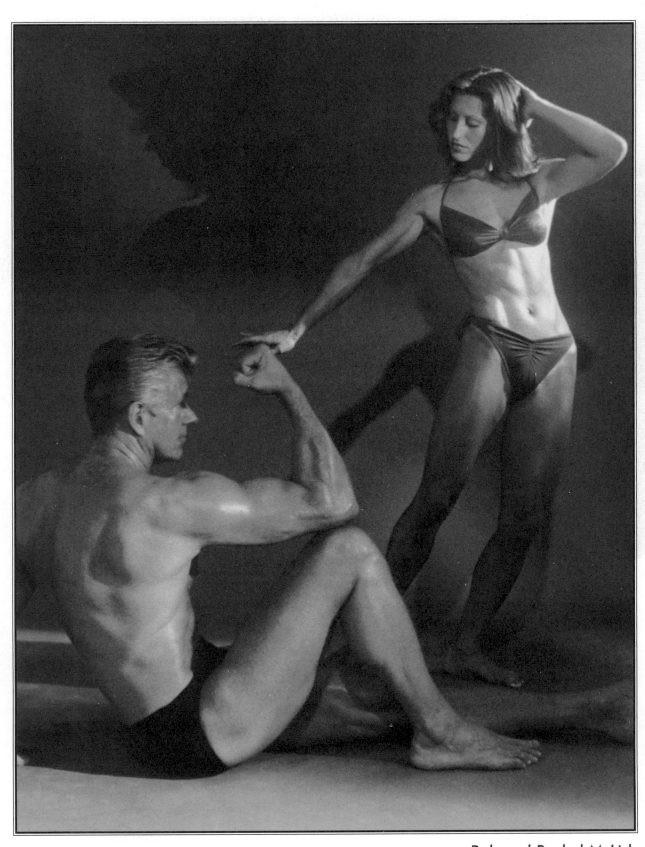

Bob and Rachel McLish

heroes in the health field, and even though Bob was of a similar age he always looked younger. In 1995 I was training Steve Collins to become the World Super-Middle-Weight Boxing Champion. On the wall there was a huge picture of Bob in his 70's looking in unbelievable shape. Steve and I just stared at this picture in disbelief. I resolved to go to California, meet with this man, discover his secrets and make them available to the world.

Frankly, when I met with Bob the following year I expected to be disappointed. Surely, he couldn't look as good as his pictures. To my delight, in the flesh he looked even better! Indeed, I will make no secret of the fact that Bob went on to become one of my heroes.

Grow Younger As You Grow Older.

He told me how, at 65, he had felt he was going downhill and had wondered what he could do about it. Bob had spent a lifetime in the health field.

He decided that he would make use of all that he learned and would attempt to do the impossible. Could he grow younger as he grew older and therefore defy the aging process? It had never been done before but if he could make such a breakthrough then he could make the pattern available to every person on the planet who wanted it.

Bob showed me the pictures of himself at 65 and then 77 and the difference was remarkable! What really impressed me about Bob was that he was a man who actually believed that growing older was a decision and that he had the secrets to reversing the process. He passionately wanted to make the secrets available to everyone. This gave him the drive and passion to continually be open to the new.

The Real Deal.

The more time I spent with Bob the more I was convinced that he was the real deal. Initially, one is struck by his impossible tan, his almost too perfect head of hair and how the sun practically glints off his teeth and muscles. But I was soon to learn that he was no paper tiger.

I arranged for him to come to Ireland and to be put through a series of tests in the top clinic in the country. The results were that Bob was one of the fittest people that they had ever tested, with a fitness level of a 25 year old.

As a body-builder that had won 12 titles, I was no stranger to weight-training. In one of my first workouts with Bob, at the end of a gruelling 1-hour session, he finished off with a bench press of 300 lbs. I remember laughing with people who had witnessed this display and saying 'Who is this guy? Superman's grandfather?' More and more I began to see the man as a pioneer, a Peter Pan who refused to grow old, who above anything wanted to extend these benefits to others, make them available to all who wanted it.

Soon, I found myself caught up in Bob's momentum and helping in any way I could. Working together we produced two videos entitled 'Secrets to Lifelong Fitness' in which Bob attempted to put everything he learned onto these tapes. He hopes at a future date to bring out a totally new book entitled 'How I Grew Younger as I Grew Older'.

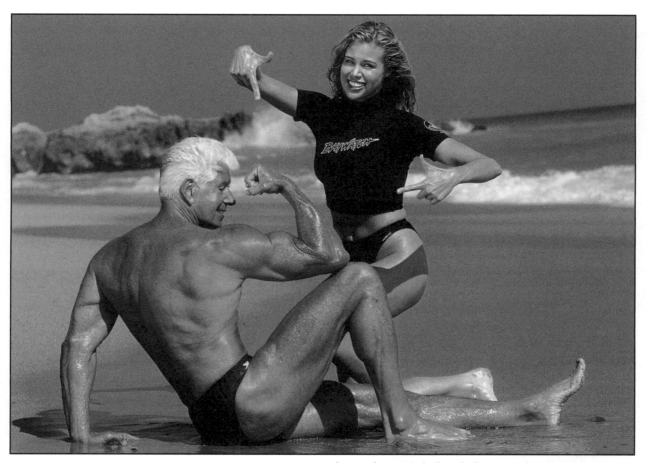

Bob on his 80th birthday, with Brooke Burns

Use More of Your Mind.

Personally, one of my life-long interests is in how to use more of your mind and apply it to every area of your life, in short, mind over matter. I've encompassed what I've learned in a system called Educo™, a Latin word which means to draw out from within. The system enables you to use more of your mind, you draw out the life and the lifestyle that you want from within. Educo™ has been the subject of 10 years research with a university in London, England. This system was also used by Steve Collins to win two world championship belts for the Super-Middle-Weight Boxing Title.

Steve, who hadn't fought in many years was able to come back and use Educo™, which enabled him to change his entire boxing style in a week (much to the astonishment of the press and then was able to fight flat out for 12 rounds and not feel tired, in addition, he could stop pain and bleeding. Steve, in his first bout beat Chris Eubank (who had had 43 fights in a row without a defeat), for the world title.

Another study carried out under university research conditions shocked even Bob, where mind over matter was applied to fat-loss. The average result was that each individual experienced an almost 12 lb difference in 12 days, losing almost 8 lbs of fat and gaining almost 3 lbs of muscle. This result would literally transform the average person's body and was achieved without a reduction in food calories, using only weight training and the power of the mind. To date, this has been the most effective weight-loss study under research conditions ever.

Bob's Biggest Breakthrough.

The main reason for this particular book is to reveal what Bob considers to be his biggest breakthrough to date. In addition to the university research, for many years I have helped people to use more of their mind for healing, health, body sculpture and rejuvenation. When I approached Bob with the possibility that using more of his mind could be the next step that he was looking for, he jumped at the opportunity. He agreed to attend one of my seminars. During the seminar he learned how to mentally relax all stress, tension, worry, problems, fears, phobias, negative thoughts, etc.

What the majority of people don't realize is that the life force, the energy within the body, often called Ki or Chi, is tied up by the mental effort that the average person puts themselves through. When you cease all effort then for the first time ever you can palpably begin to feel the body's uncovered and freed energy. This seems to emanate from the area of the Solar Plexus, rather like electricity and moves upward to the head where it is often seen as a bright white light, runs down the arms and the legs. In the process, the person becomes happy, blissful, even euphoric. The more the person is prepared to let go of the mental effort the more every single cell in the body can be filled up with energy and light.

While Bob had meditated daily for over 50 years this was the first time he experienced the freeing up of his own energy. After his first session he likened it to being reborn, that every single cell in his body was fully cleared and activated in the process. In addition, he was thrilled at how energized he felt after this process. The aim of Educo™ is to draw out your life and lifestyle from within. So, Bob started working daily with drawing out his life energy in the manner described.

Programming.

The next stage of Educo™ is drawing out your lifestyle from within. To do this it is necessary to use programming. Together, Bob and I designed a program for health, energy, strength and rejuvenation which we then attempted to install into every cell of his body and bring about results at this cellular level. To do this Bob relaxed to the point that his whole body filled up with energy and light and every single cell was activated. Then he played his mind-program from an audiotape while at this photographic-mind level. The results from the program are what prompted this book. They were so great that Bob wanted to get this information out to people quickly rather than have to wait on a new book. Bob has described this mind over matter and life as a pyramid where he puts the Educo™ System at the top and it effects everything else in a cascade effect. To quote Bob, 'If I were to take all of my secrets and I could only avail of one then it would have to be using more of the mind. It comes closer to being THE answer than anything else I've discovered.'

Human Computer Programming.
How to program your mind for the goals that you want.

Let me begin by saying that my Master of Science Degree is in this area and most of the results I attained with people came from giving them programs. Because you are reading this, I can presuming that you would like to enact a program in one or more of the following areas; fat-loss, body-sculpture, health, rejuvenation, happiness, success etc. You need to make up your mind, photograph your goal, and imprint it on your unconscious/subconscious. Then it becomes far easier or even effortless to achieve your goals.

To understand how your mind works, consider an iceberg. When we see an iceberg we know that what we see above the water is only a small percentage of what is below the water. The part of the iceberg that we can see above the water is the conscious mind and that below the water is the unconscious or subconscious mind. To achieve successful programming, we need to get the WHOLE mind totally focused on the goal to the exclusion of all opposing doubts. In other words we must fill our mind with ONLY with our goal. The vital word here is WHOLE mind, the conscious and the subconscious.

Let me give you an example. Suppose you have very little money and your goal is to make a million. In most cases we would say that your wish is to make a million. Why? Because it will depend on the percentage of your mind that thinks that the goal is possible. Therefore, if you say, 'I want to make a million,' what percentage of your mind says, 'I can't really see that happening'? With doubt programming is negated and won't reach your unconscious mind. In turn your unconscious mind, being the greater percentage of your mind, is not activated by the programming. At the best a small percentage of your positive goal reaches your unconscious, which is not enough to achieve your outcome. It is vital that you understand this explanation. If you liken your mind to having 1,000 employees, then you have interested only a few in carrying our your task. What is necessary is to interest ALL of the them carrying out the task. The simplest way to do this is to come up with a big goal. A big goal about which you can become so excited that logic and opposing thoughts are negated by passion and excitement.

The recipe for failure is to come up with a small goal that only interests a few of those "employees". You have to start with a goal that's literally so exciting that it should propel you out of bed in the morning. After all, if it's not a big, exciting, life-changing goal then why do you want it? If you want to discover the possibilities of this approach you need a BIG goal. In essence, what you are doing is catching all of the attention of your WHOLE mind with the end product or outcome that you want to achieve. For the short period of time that you're imprinting the program you need to suspend so-called logic or disbelief.

Just think of yourself as a director of the perfect mental movie. You are now going to sit down and write out a very brief script based on the outcome you desire. Then you transfer that mental movie to an audiotape. Then you play it to yourself while filling all of your mind with this mental program.

This is exactly how Bob and I designed his program. First of all, write down your end product. This is then divided into three sections, visual, auditory and kinesthetic (feeling). In Bob's case it was "What would I look like when I achieve my goal"? Every single cell of his body would be lit up with energy and light. He would be this picture of glowing health. He would look years younger than his actual age, perfect tan, perfect teeth, full head of white hair, body-sculptured to perfection. See yourself as a sculptor and now see that perfect creation in your mind.

You would see yourself with people and they would look at you in stunned awe, in disbelief. Have fun, go for it, see yourself as the healthiest person on the planet.

See yourself leading groups of people back to youth. See them getting younger as you are speaking to them. Picture yourself taking them up to a fork in the road where on one side it says 'Age' and on the other side 'Youth' and as you're leading them off on the youthful side they are becoming younger and younger. (Exaggerate it, having them throwing away sticks, straightening up and becoming exuberant) See yourself then inspiring rooms-full of people, maybe even TV audiences and really making a difference. Remember, you need to catch all of the attention of your mind with your mental program. So, just dwell on all of the positives, get totally caught up in it.

Auditory.

Now write out the auditory side. Hear yourself telling others that to grow old is just a decision and to grow young is also a decision. Have your voice filled with certainty. Hear yourself explain to people how you understood that you must have a goal that's so big that all of the workers in your mind want it. Have people clapping and cheering you enthusiastically, more excited than ever before. You'd be shouting it from the rooftops, so, when you're listening to your own voice in the program make it really excited, passionate. Writing down this program and focusing your mind on it is an integral part of the programming process. Imagine achieving such an outcome and how excited you will be. You would have cracked one of the great belief systems of humanity. So let your voice take on that kind of excitement.

Kinesthetic.

Now, write down how you would feel about all of this. You'd be so excited, happy, free. Every single cell in your body and mind would be more fully alive than ever before. Get the feeling of what it would be like to talk to individuals and groups of people and pump them up, the hope and the possibility of a more youthful future. Get those feelings and see people more inspired and excited than ever before.

Participation and Emotional Intensity.

Ideally, think of yourself as an actor or actress who is really participating in your new role. You are so excited about this new role that you're giving all of the emotional intensity that you can muster. Do anything that makes it more real for you. When you act out the part you involve all of your mind. So if cheering, jumping up and down, smiling, clapping, various actions are required, do them. Do whatever it takes.

Remember, to achieve your big goal you must allow it to happen. Going back to Bob, he was able, using programming, to convince himself that it was possible. That's all you need to do, to convince your own mind. No one knows what is truly possible in any area until they try. The great adventure is to find out.

The next step is to get an audiotape and record your program. Remember to speak somewhat faster than normal and with as much enthusiasm and certainty as possible and in a voice tone that conveys the idea that this is already done. Ideally the program should run for no less than 20 minutes but no longer than 40.

Stop and consider.

This is the most important thing you have ever done in your life – so do it perfectly.

Play your program at least once daily. When you have played it for over a month, it will have the added bonus of a conditioning effect. You should never play your tape while driving your car or operating any machine or anything that requires your full attention. You should be in a quiet place, preferably relaxed, either sitting or lying down, and when the tape is playing, fill your entire mind with it. Participate and go along with the actions. Ideally act it out and make it totally real.

Further Hints.

Visual: make everything as big and bright as possible. The bigger you make things the more impact they have on the mind. Make the picture 10 times normal size. The whole scene should be extra colorful. Make the picture perfect for you.

Sound: make the sound perfect for you, put in whatever background sounds or noises you would like to make it perfect - generate as much excitement, interest, certainty in all of the voices. Clapping and cheering may help.

Feeling: include extra feelings to make it perfect. These may be feelings of heat, breeze, being clapped on the back, handshakes or other external feelings to achieve reality.

Taste: in some situations taste will aid results. There may be champagne, salt air, celebratory dinner, chocolates etc.

Smells: may help the reality. There could be sea air, food,champagne, aftershave, perfume etc.

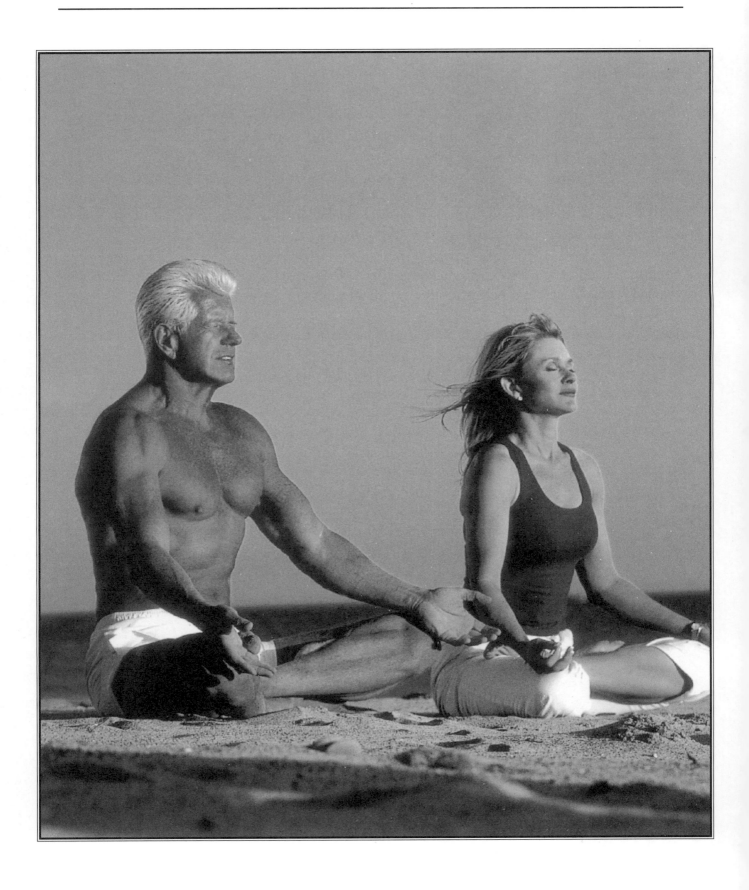

Breathing

Attitude Breathing™
A tool from HeartMath®

Researchers at the famous Institute of HeartMath in Boulder Creek, California have found that the human heart incorporates more than 40,000 neurons that form an "intelligence" that can be used to fight the effects of stress. For example, the proliferation of core emotions associated with the heart (such as love appreciation and care) increases the activity of the parasympathetic nervous system, slowing the body's heart rate and relaxing its internal systems. In addition, the Institute of HeartMath recommends employing a "Attitude Breathing Technique" in stressful situations. At the core of this stress management technique is the concept that stress is nothing more than a matter of perception. The more you practice it the more helpful it becomes.

Attitude Breathing™ is especially useful for calming yourself when feeling anxious. Attitude Breathing helps to soothe and disperse anxious feelings, bringing you back into balance.

Step 1. Shift your attention to your heart and solar plexus/stomach area.

Step 2. Ask yourself, "What would be a better attitude for me to maintain in this situation?" Then, set up an inner attitude, like "stay calm", "stay neutral in this situation", "don't judge before you know the facts", "make peace with this", or decide what attitude is appropriate for your situation.

Step 3. Next, gently and sincerely pretend to breathe the new attitude you want in through the heart. Then breathe it out through the solar plexus and stomach to anchor it. Do this for a while until you feel the new attitude has set in.

Use Attitude Breathing™ to help release tension in any part of the body. As you do this, ask yourself, "What would be a more balanced feeling or approach to what I'm doing?" Once you feel more emotionally balanced, then pretend to breathe the feeling of balance through the area of tension. You'll start to feel the tension release as more of your balanced heart energy moves through that area. Attitude Breathing is especially useful for calming yourself when you feel anxiety - or before entering a situation that usually makes you feel anxious (before a business meeting, before traveling or before a new social encounter, for example). Using Attitude Breathing helps soothe and disperse the anxious feelings and brings you back to balance.

Stopping emotional reactivity: During stressful times, many people are experiencing more negative emotions, such as anxiety, fear, uncertainty, grief, and anger. This can make us more edgy and irritable and sometimes cause us to react strongly to others before we think twice about it. At times, you might notice this kind of emotional reactivity in yourself or in those around you, including your co-workers, friends, or family. When you feel yourself beginning to react emotionally to someone or something, use Attitude Breathing to take the excess negative emotion out of your reaction. Anchoring your energy in your heart and solar plexus will help you stay centered and see calmly and clearly how best to respond.

This and other techniques for facilitating emotional clarity and optimal performance are outlined in Doctor Childres' and Howard Martin's empowering book *The Heart Math Solution*. I took their course at the Institute of HeartMath a few years ago and have relied on, and incorporated into my daily routine, their techniques even since.

How to Breathe During Exercise

Unlike Attitude Breathing which is done for relaxation or calming, you also need to learn how to breathe properly during exercise.

Every day breathing is done in and out through the nose. During exercise, when a greater volume of air is required by the body, it is acceptable to breathe through the mouth. However there is a more powerful way to breathe while you exercise. This is called Throat Breathing or Swedish Breathing. First become aware of the appropriate muscles by clearing your throat. Consciously feel the muscles specifically being used. Next say the word "Who" so it sounds like a soft 'whoosh' and extend the second silent 'W'. Extend the 'W' continuously so you can feel the air rushing from your mouth. The sensation you feel in the throat indicates which muscles you need to used during throat breathing. Once you are aware of the appropriate muscles, perform an exhalation using the throat.

In addition to the above you also need to learn to breathe from your abdomen. Normally you inhale and exhale by expanding your ribcage, but this type of breathing is very shallow and takes in little oxygen. When you exercise, you need to greatly increase the amount of oxygen to the bloodstream and the best way to do that is to breathe with your abdomen.

When you begin to inhale, draw out your diaphragm and expand the abdomen - exhaling involves pulling the abdomen in so that the belly button moves toward the spine as the air is expelled. It may look a little silly, but you will feel right away how much more oxygen you are inhaling.

Now combine abdomen breathing with throat breathing; this is the most efficient way to breathe during medium or heavy exercise.

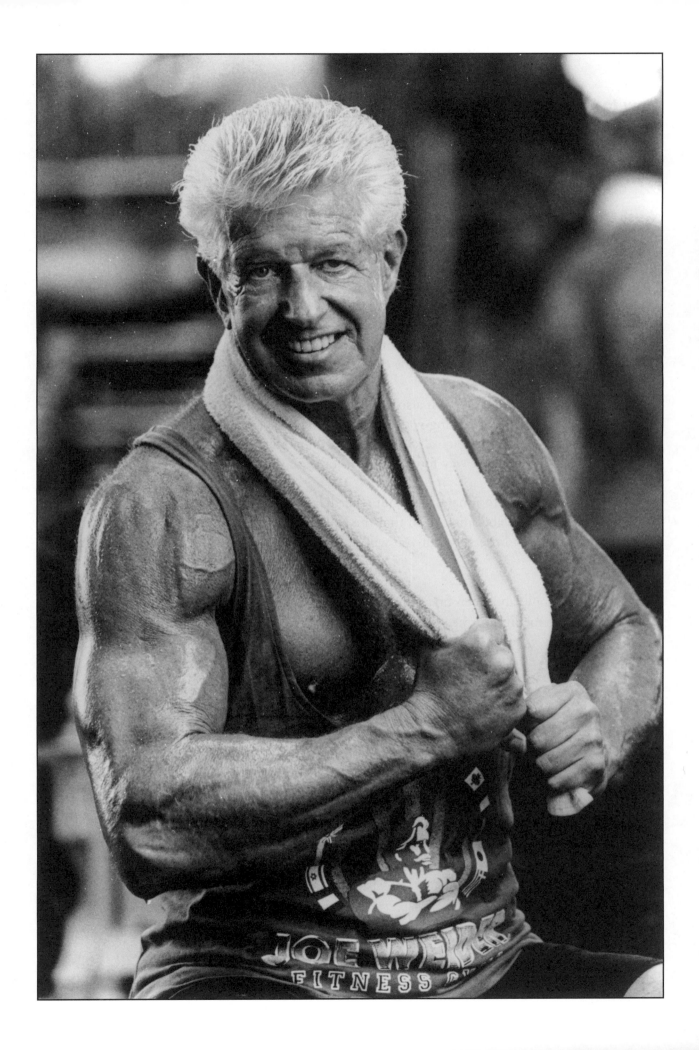

Phase One: The Warm Up

Every workout should begin with a warm-up and stretching routine. I can't stress this enough. Aerobic exercises and strength training are important to good health, but flexibility is the key to your independence and coordination, and to the prevention of injuries. It's also part of the American College of Sports Medicine's statement on minimum fitness. Stiffness can start as early as our thirties and will only worsen with each advancing year. But this decline is reversible. With the proper flexibility exercises, even men and women with restricted mobility will see noticeable improvements.

Tight joints and muscles are typically the result of inactivity — you lose the motions you do not use. Stretching loosens this tightness, lubricating the joints and allowing you to work each muscle through its full range of motion. Most important, staying limber also means you're able to continue enjoying your normal activities — well into the golden years. It is a must that you have all of the below as you age.

Regular stretching will accomplish the following:

- Reduce muscle tension
- Prevent muscle and joint injuries
- Improve circulation
- Improve balance and flexibility
- Improve coordination and agility
- Increase range of motion
- Strengthen your tendons, ligaments and muscles

45

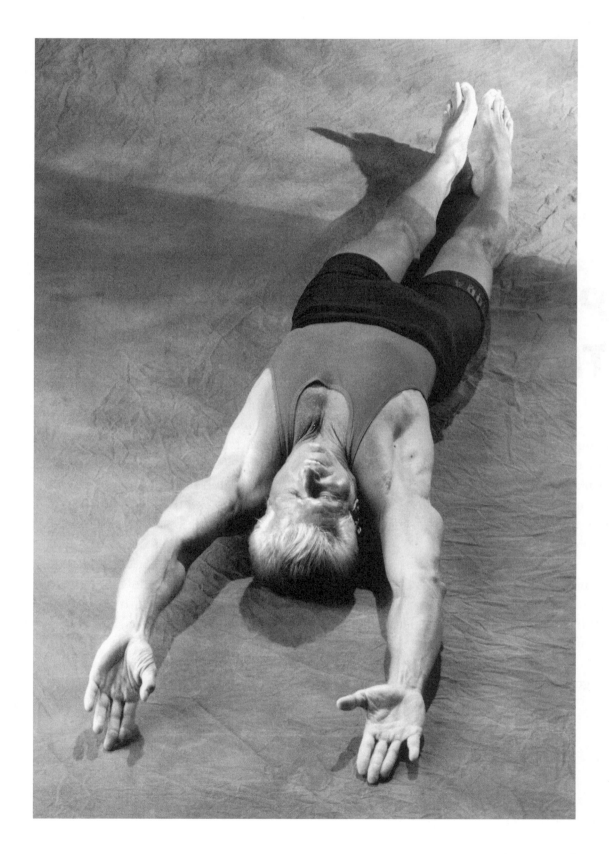

The Sprawl

You should start each stretching routine by taking it slowly, especially in the beginning. You might find some of the stretches uncomfortable at first, because you'll be working muscles you forgot you had. Give yourself time to adjust to the stress and strain. Stretching is not a competitive sport — you don't have to beat the clock or an opponent to gain an advantage. Enjoy the exercise by learning how to stretch properly and effectively. Stretch your muscles and joints only to a point of tension. Flexibility exercises should always be done in a slow, controlled movement.jerky movements will only cause pain and injury. If it hurts, stop.

It bears repeating: The correct technique is to relax and sustain the tension while focusing your attention on the muscles being stretched; the improper method is to bounce up and down, or to stretch to the point of pain.

Begin each session with a five minute walk, just to warm up your muscles, then move on to an easy stretch. Go to the point where you feel a mild stretch of the muscles, and relax. The feeling of tension should subside as you hold the position. If it does not, ease off slightly and find a degree of tension that is comfortable. Learn to respect your body's signals.

After the easy stretch, move slowly into a more extreme stretch. Move a fraction of an inch farther until you again feel that stretch and hold for 5 to 30 seconds. Be in control. The tension should diminish. If it does not, again ease off slightly. Breathing should be slow and relaxed. Perform the movement as you exhale, and breathe slowly as you hold your stretch.

Once you learn how to stretch, you'll be able to develop your own routines to suit your individual needs, but in the following pages I'm going to show you the stretches I use before and after my workouts.

A lot of people don't stretch because they think it's pointless. As a result, they push themselves too hard and too quickly and wind up with an injury. I stretch because I want to be sure that my tendons, ligaments, and muscles are loose and flexible. That's why I've never had a muscle strain or pull.

I recommend at least 6 to 10 stretches every morning, whether you're working out or not. Perform each exercise 3 to 6 times. Try to pick one stretch for each major muscle group (my favorites are listed at the end of this chapter). If I'm feeling particularly tight, sore, or tense during the day, I pull out a few of my favorites in the evening and stretch to relieve my tension.

(Note: Be sure to consult your physician before beginning any stretching or exercise program, particularly if you've been inactive for a long time.)

The Sprawl

Lie on your back with your arms overhead, pointing north, and your feet pointing south. Stretch your arms, shoulders, spine, abdominal muscles, feet, and ankles by reaching with your hands and pointing with your toes, as if you were being pulled in two different directions. Try pulling in your abdominal muscles with each stretch.This is a great exercise to start the morning.

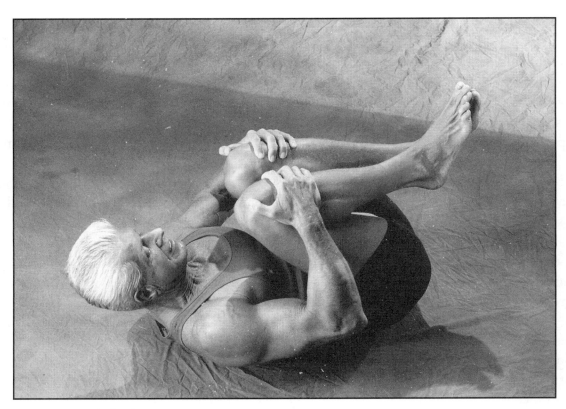

Two-Legged Curl

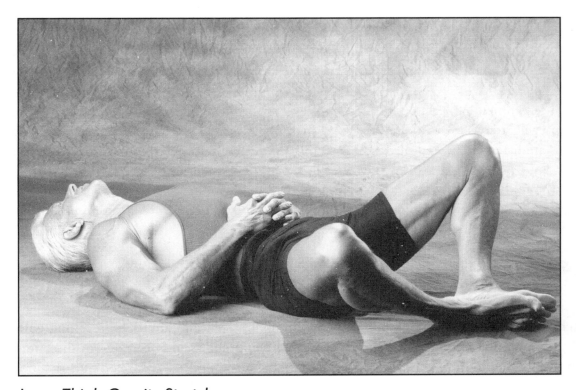

Inner Thigh Gravity Stretch

One-Legged Curl

While still on your back, bend one knee and gently pull it toward your chest to stretch the lower back and leg. Keep your head on the floor, if possible. Don't forget to stretch the other side.

Two-Legged Curl

After pulling one leg at a time to your chest, pull both legs to your chest. Concentrate on curling your head up toward your knees.

Lower-Back Stretch

Lie on your back, with your knees bent, feet flat on the floor, and hands behind your head. Tighten your butt and abdominal muscles to relieve the tension in your lower back. Hold for several seconds, then relax. Next, move your arms flat along the sides of your body, take a deep breath, and slowly raise your trunk off the floor. Slowly exhale and lower your body back to the floor.

Neck Stretch

From the starting position of the last stretch, turn your chin toward your right shoulder, keeping your head to the floor. Turn your chin only to the point of an easy stretch. Hold, then stretch to the other side.

The Crunch

Beginning from the same position, only with your fingers interlaced behind your head — as if you were going to do a sit-up — slowly pull your head forward until you feel a slight stretch in the back of the neck. Hold for several seconds, then lower your head back to the floor. This exercise helps reduce tension in the neck and upper-spine areas, where headaches often originate.

Inner-Thigh Gravity Stretch

While still on your back, place the soles of your feet together and allow gravity to pull your knees apart, stretching the inner thigh and groin areas. Hold for several seconds, and relax.

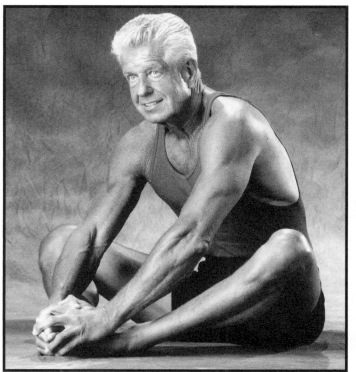

Sitting Inner-Thigh Stretch

Sitting Hamstring Stretch

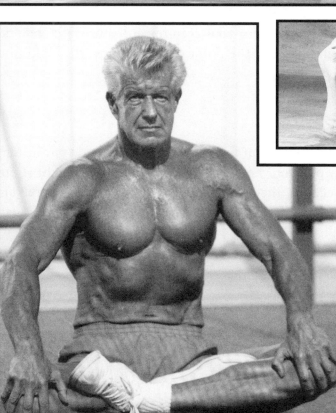

The Lotus

Sitting Inner-Thigh Stretch

While sitting on the floor, place the soles of your feet together much as you did in the last exercise. Bring your heels to a comfortable distance from your crotch. Grab your feet and toes with both hands and gently pull your upper body forward to again feel an easy stretch in the inner thigh and groin areas. Do not bend forward from your neck. Begin the move from your hips, keeping your lower back flat and your eyes looking straight ahead. Hold for several seconds, if possible, without strain, and then release. Keep your elbows on or near your knees to help enhance the stretch. Once the tension has diminished, increase the stretch by gently pulling yourself forward even more.

Sitting Hamstring Stretch

You've seen this stretch before. Runners often use it to stretch the hamstrings, the group of tendons at the back of the knees. Straighten the left leg and tuck the right leg up next to you so that the sole of the right foot is facing the inside of the left upper thigh. Do not "lock" the straight leg. Stretch the upper-left hamstrings by gently bending forward from your hips, with your foot upright, toes and ankle relaxed, eyes straight ahead. Use a towel, if necessary — it will help you keep the stretch. Grasp the ends and wrap the towel around your foot. Bring your torso forward by pulling on the towel, using your foot as a brace. Then stretch the other side.

The Lotus

This particular Yoga stretch has no real value other than serving as a great stress-buster. Some people can easily assume this position while others can't. If it hurts, don't push it. And be sure to work through the first position before moving on to the second.

Sit on the floor with both legs extended. Using both hands, place your left foot high on your right thigh. Your knee should remain on the floor (make sure you loosen up your ankles first). If it doesn't, do not proceed to the next step until you've mastered this one. It may take you many weeks of stretching before you can assume this position. Once you have, bend your right knee and place your right foot high on the left thigh by sliding it along the left leg. Keep your back straight. You're now in the full lotus position. Breathe deeply and relax.

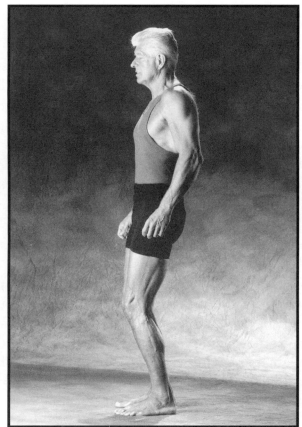

Standing Hamstring Stretch

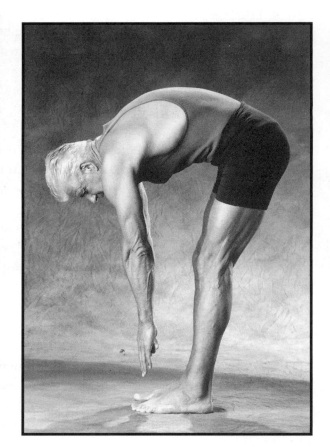

The Toe Touch

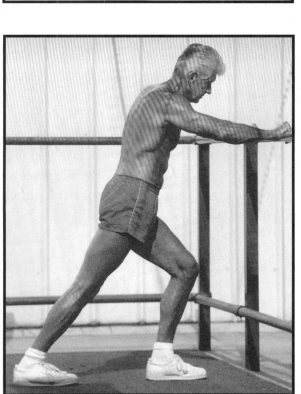

Standing Calf Stretch

Standing Hamstring Stretch

Stand with your feet about shoulder-width apart and pointed straight ahead, and keep your back straight. Bend your knees slightly to tighten the quadriceps, the muscles on the front of your thighs, and to relax and stretch the hamstrings. If you're doing this exercise correctly, the quadriceps should feel hard and tight, the hamstrings soft and relaxed while being stretched.

The Toe Touch

From the starting position of the last stretch, slowly bend forward from the hips, as if you're trying to touch your toes. Keep your knees slightly bent to avoid stress on the lower back. Let your neck and arms relax to the point where you feel a slight stretch in the lower back, hips, groin, and hamstrings. Hold this position for several seconds until you're relaxed. Some of you may even be able to touch your toes.

Step 'n' Stretch

Place the ball of one foot on the edge of a staircase, with your heel hanging over the edge. Lower your heel below the level of the stair to stretch your Achilles tendon and ankle. Keep your leg straight. Hold on to the railing for balance. Do not bounce.

Standing Calf Stretch

Stand at arms length away from a wall or support rail and lean on it with your hands. Bend your front leg and straighten the other leg behind you, keeping both feet flat on the floor. Slowly move your hips forward to stretch the legs and hips. Switch positions and work it again. This is a great exercise for walkers and joggers.

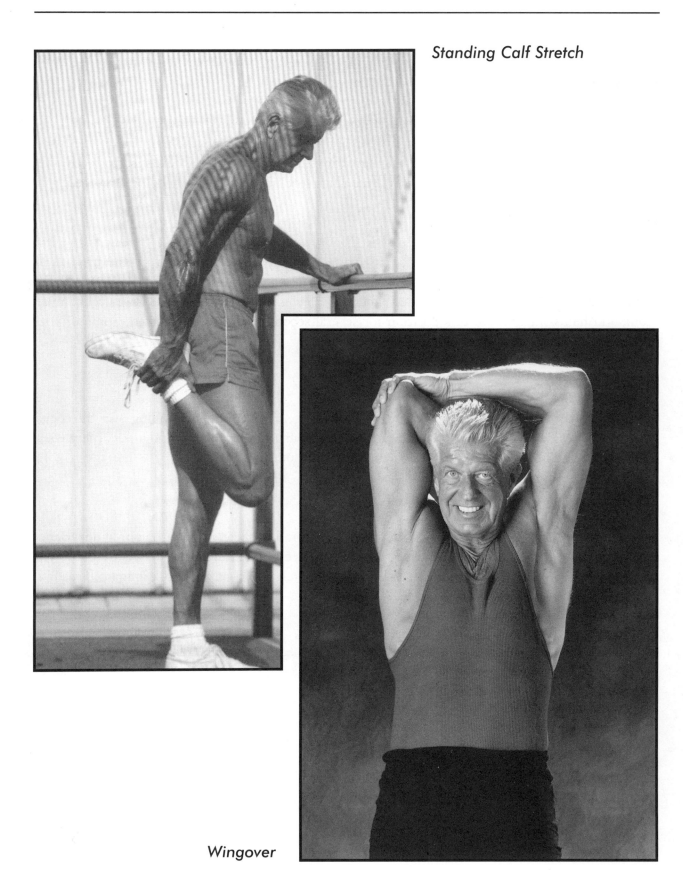

Standing Calf Stretch

Wingover

Standing Quad Stretch

While still leaning against a wall or support rail, use your right hand to hold the top of your right foot behind you. Gently pull your heel up to your buttocks to stretch the knee and quadriceps. The knee should bend naturally. Hold for several seconds, then stretch the other leg.

Wingover

Raise your arms overhead and hold your right elbow with your left hand. Allow your right hand to dangle behind your neck. Gently pull your elbow behind your head to stretch your triceps (the muscles along the back of your upper arms) and the top of your shoulders. Hold for several seconds and release, then stretch the other side.

Deep Breathing

This one is not really a stretch, but the additional oxygen it provides will do wonders for your vitality. Breathe deeply, swelling your lower abdomen to its fullest, like a baby lying on its back – then exhale slowly returning you stomach to normal. Repeat several times. If you see spots in front of your eyes or if you feel faint, stop and relax. As you get used to the rush of oxygen entering your system the spots will slowly disappear. You can perform this exercise throughout the day — while driving, at your desk, or in bed. It's great as a pick-me-up or use it to relax.

My Favorite Stretches

- The Sprawl, for the entire body
- Lower-Back Stretch, for the lower back
- Sitting Inner-Thigh Stretch, for the inner thighs and groin
- Sitting Hamstring Stretch, for the hamstrings
- Standing Calf Stretch, for the calf muscles
- Wingover, for the triceps and shoulders
- Deep breathing, for vitality and energy

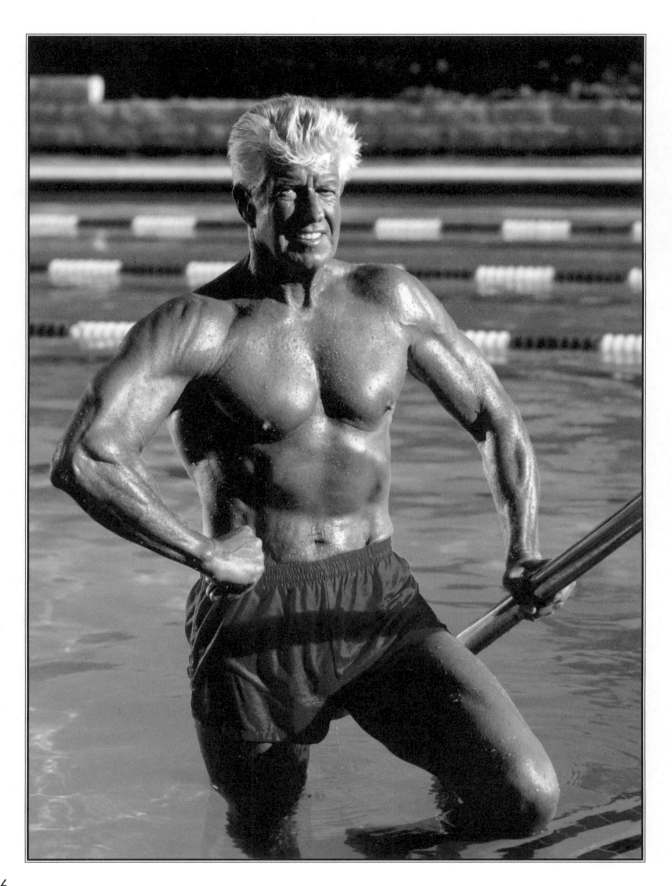

Phase Two:
The IsoTension Program

My IsoTension program was developed over 60 years ago during a period of my life when I just couldn't make it to the gym. I put together a series of exercises that provides just the right combination of isometrics, isotonics and resistance training. It takes only several minutes to perform each one, and the results after several weeks will astound you. You'll not only increase the size and strength of your muscles, but you'll also realize other benefits that go far beyond what was once believed possible by experts in the health and fitness industry. For example, as recently reported by the Arthritis Foundation, isometric exercises and other gentle movements of the joints can help arthritis by improving muscle strength around the joints and maintaining range of motion. When you improve the strength of the muscles around your joints you're actually improving the strength of your joint because it can withstand greater stress.

Isotonic exercises are those that contract a set of muscles, often while you're moving a joint. Isometric exercises involve working a set of muscles against an immovable object, changing only the tension. By using both techniques, you'll work your muscles to their full range of motion, which allows blood to continue flowing to the working muscles. Remember, it's imperative to take each movement to its fullest extension. And never hold your breath. It tends to cause a rise in your blood pressure. Proper breathing will enable you to do more work with less fatigue.

IsoTension alone will not affect your body weight, increase your stamina, or condition your cardiovascular system. But it's a great way to get you pumped, to improve your muscle tone, and to ready you for the intermediate and more advanced stages of weight training (Chapter Eight).

Even if you're a bodybuilder or weight lifter, you can use this method of training as a complement to your regular program. All the exercises found in this chapter help round out and develop the form of your muscles. Hard-core bodybuilders, especially, often use a few of these exercises to "peak out" their muscles before a show or contest. I've put bodybuilders, weekend athletes, and men and women in their thirties, fifties, and eighties on my IsoTension program, and all of them have experienced a noticeable difference in their mental attitude, their energy, and their bodies — with a minimum of effort. So will you.

The basic principle for the following series of exercises is that if you simply cause the muscle to work against another object, causing it to tense to its utmost, the muscle will automatically be strengthened. No motion is wasted. All you'll use is an ordinary bath towel and your own opposing strength. This makes it an especially valuable routine for those of you who travel a lot and can't always make it to the gym. I've been known to exercise in hotel rooms, even on airplanes. Wherever it's possible to push or pull by using your own strength, you'll know you're never far from maintaining your health.

Muscles are built on the negative, not the positive. When you're doing a push-up, for example, the muscle gets completely taxed on the downward (or negative) motion, not on the actual "push up" itself. If you do only the "push up" portion of the exercise, you end up working only 75 to 80 percent of the muscle. You must concentrate on the "negative" motion in order to exert the muscle to its fullest. All exercises should be done with proper form, total concentration, and balance, otherwise you're wasting your time.

I've listed my suggestions for beginning your own IsoTension program at the end of this chapter. The entire routine should take you no more than 45 to 50 minutes every other day — surely a small price to pay for your health. I've used this routine consistently for 50 years, and if I had to choose only one fitness routine, this is the one I'd do.

Shoulder Press

Grasp the opposite ends of a towel in each hand and hold it behind you so that your left forearm is across the small of your back and your right arm is held up, with the elbow bent. Resisting with your left arm, push the towel upward with your right hand until it is straight up in the air. Resisting with your right arm, pull downward with your left hand until you've returned to the starting position. This builds the shoulder muscles. Switch the position of your hands, so that the right hand is behind your back and your left arm is away from your shoulder. Repeat the exercise. Keeping correct form an rhythm is important in this exercise.

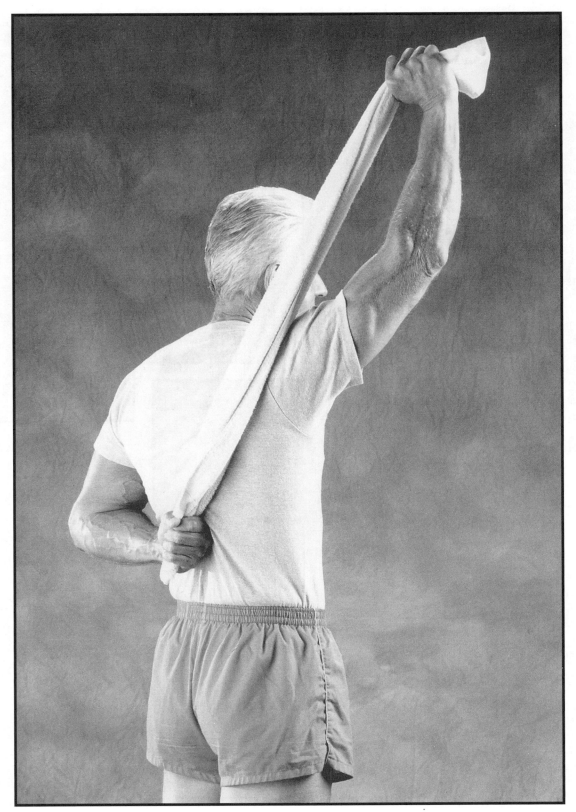

Shoulder Press

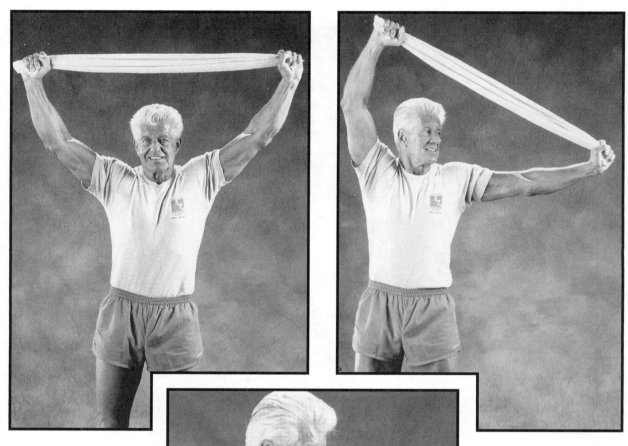

Shoulder Swing

Shoulder Swing

Tug-Away

Shoulder Swing

Grip the towel with your hands about 2 1/2 feet apart. Keeping your arms rigid, raise the towel straight above your head. Resisting forcefully with your right arm, pull with your left arm until your right biceps touches your head. Begin tugging the other way, to the right, still keeping up the opposing pressure until your left biceps touches your head. This exercise will help build your deltoid muscles, the large triangular muscles that cover the shoulder joints, as well as the trapezius muscles on the upper part of your back. It also gives you better posture, which makes you look taller. Remember: This exercise should be done slowly, and the amount of force exerted by one arm against the other should be equal.

Tug-Away

Loop a towel around a doorknob or something secure like a stair rail (or use a partner, if you have one). Grasp the ends of your towel with both hands, like a grip on a baseball bat, and stand with your feet spread slightly more than shoulder width apart, and with your knees bent. Pull your body toward the door using the towel, then slowly let your body return to the original position. This exercise helps build the latissimus dorsi — otherwise known as the lats — which are the muscles at the outside edge of your shoulder blades that develop that V-shape in your back. As you move your body to and from the door, maintain a steady tug on the towel throughout the exercise.

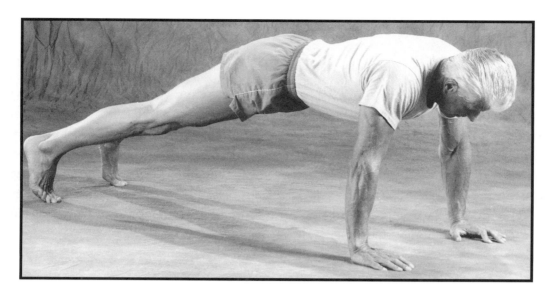

Push-Up

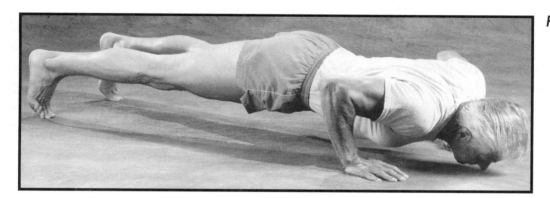

Push-Up

Push-Up from Knees

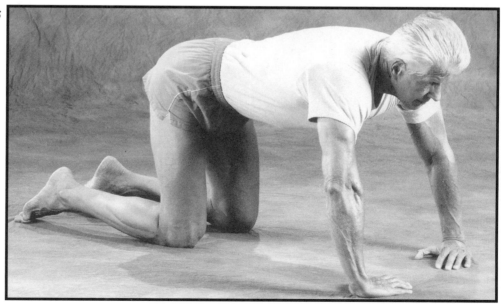

Push-Up

Lie on your stomach with your feet braced against the wall or a heavy piece of furniture. Place the palms of your hands on the floor near your shoulders and push yourself up to arms length, keeping your legs straight and your hips at all times slightly higher than your shoulders. Lower your body until your chin is within 2 or 3 inches of the floor and push up again.

The ideal form is to keep the body as one unit from heels to shoulders. If you need a little help, try doing the push-up from your knees. Those who want a more strenuous workout should use chairs or some other type of support. Set the chairs about shoulder width apart and place the palms of your hands on the seats. Push yourself to arms length and then lower your body until your chin falls below the seat level. This is a great exercise for toning and building the pectoral muscles.

Push-Up from Knees

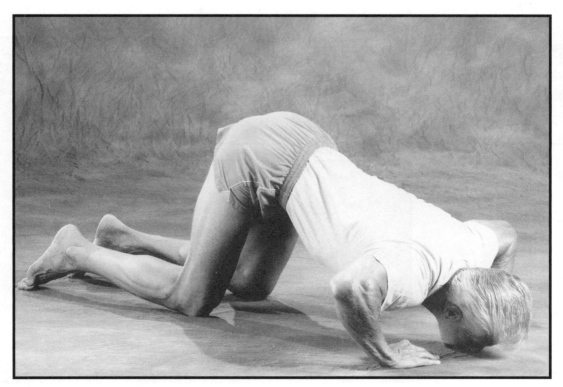

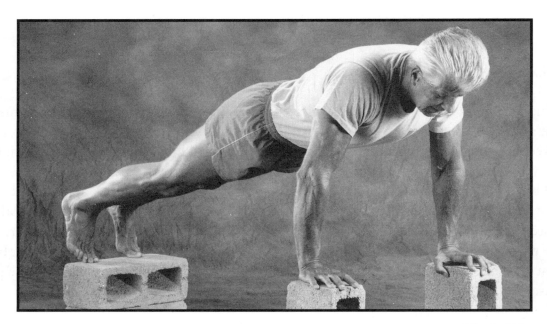

Chair Dip

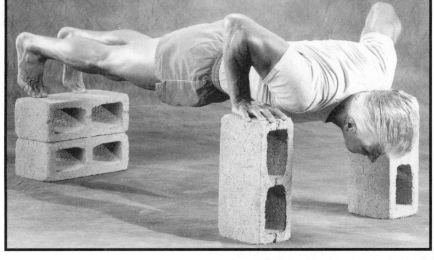

Chair Dip

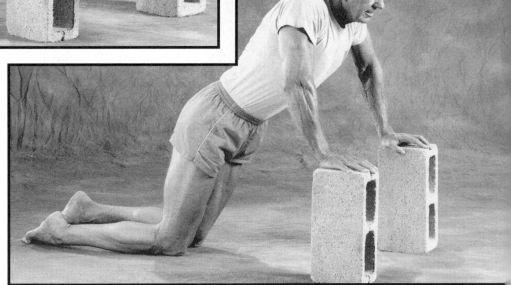

Chair Dip from Knees

Chair Dip

Place two straight-back chairs (or bricks) face to face and slightly more than shoulder width apart. With your body facing down, place the palms of your hands not far from the edge. Your palms should be firmly planted on the seats of the chairs. Caution: If they're too far forward you could slip and hurt yourself. Extend your legs behind you, keeping them straight throughout the exercise. Lower yourself until your chest dips below the seat of the chair, and push up to arms length (version 1). Similar to the push-up, this movement builds the chest, shoulders, back and arms. If you need help, try doing the Chair Dip from your knees (version 2). No bouncing. Those who want a more strenuous workout can use a low footstool to raise the feet (version 3). This is probably the single best exercise for your upper body. This exercise was the favorite of Charles Atlas and is my favorite as well, its a terrific way to build up your upper body.

Chair Dip from Knees

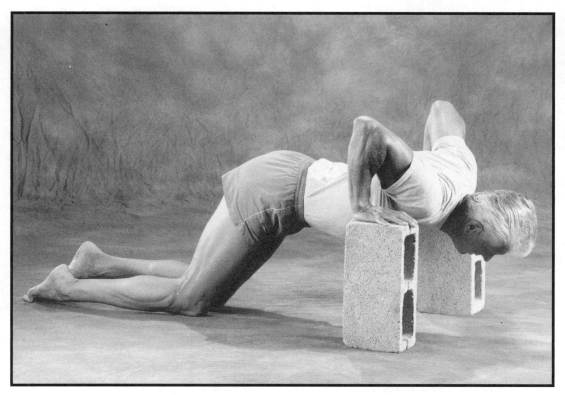

Pectoral Push

Concentration Towel Curl

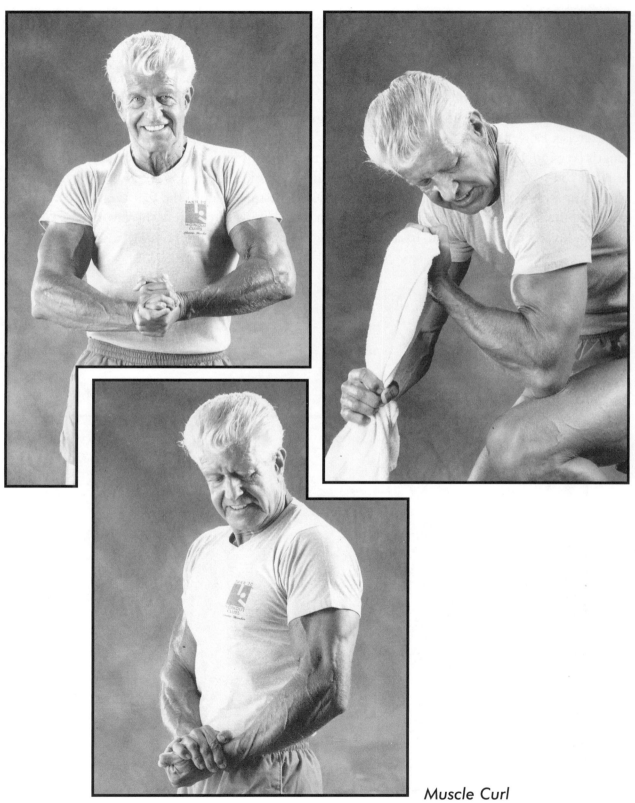

Muscle Curl

Stand with your feet shoulder width apart and clasp your hands in front of your stomach, as if you were the mother superior. Using the tension of your chest muscles, push one hand against the other with equal and opposing strength, flexing your pectoral muscles, which connect the walls of your chest to your upper arms and shoulders. This is a particularly good exercise for women, especially if they can't do the Chair Dip.

Concentration Towel Curl

In a sitting position, brace your left elbow on your left thigh near the knee. Hold both ends of a towel in your right hand and grasp the loop of the towel in your left hand, palm up. Lean forward and pull upward with your left hand while resisting with your right to work the biceps. Next pull downward with your right hand, resisting with your left. Repeat to the other side. Work the muscle to full extension and contraction, and don't bend your wrist. This exercise targets the biceps, toning and firming that area of the arm that tends to jiggle under short sleeved shirts or blouses as we get older. Be sure to work slowly and follow good rhythm and form.

Muscle Curl

Clasp your hands at waist level (with your right hand on top) and push upward with your left hand while resisting with your right. This works the biceps. After finishing a set with the left arm, switch the position of your hands and repeat the workout with the right biceps. A lot of muscle is built on the "negative" force, so be sure to concentrate on the downward movement as well.

Biceps Flex

This is the old make-a-muscle motion. Just flex your biceps to help round out the contours of the muscle. Concentrate on pumping blood to the muscle by bending your wrist inward. Hold for several seconds. Feel it tighten by slowly flexing and un-flexing the biceps to its maximum potential. After finishing with the right arm, switch positions and repeat the workout with the left biceps.

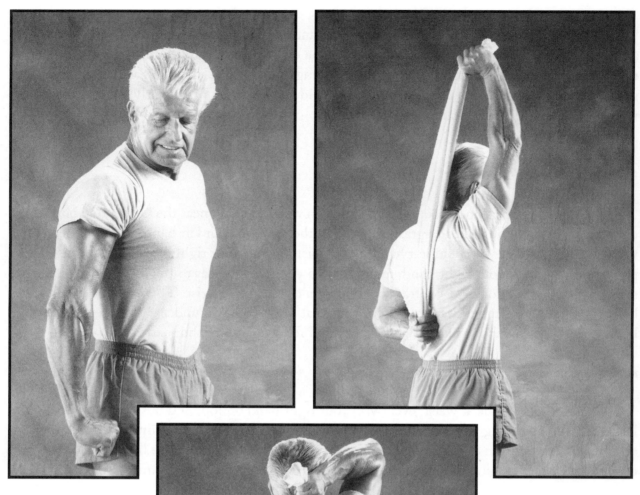

Triceps Flex

Triceps Press

Triceps Press

Triceps Flex

As with the Biceps Flex, your objective is to flex the triceps. Do this by straightening your right arm slightly behind you while concentrating on pumping blood to the muscle by turning your wrist toward your body. Feel the muscle tighten as you slowly flex and un-flex the triceps to its maximum potential. After finishing with the right arm, switch positions and repeat the workout with the left triceps. Repeat 5-10 times holding for 5-10 seconds each time.

Triceps Press

Grasp the opposite ends of a towel in each hand and hold it behind you so that your left forearm is across the small of your back and your right arm is extended straight overhead. The palm of your left hand should face away from your body as you grasp the towel. Resisting with your right arm, pull the towel downward with your left hand until your right forearm is across the back of your head and your left arm is extended straight downward. Resisting with your left arm, pull upward with your right arm in an easy rhythmic motion until you've returned to the starting position. This builds the triceps along the back of the upper arm, one of the first areas of fat deposits once we reach 30. Next, switch the position of your hands, so that the right forearm is across the small of your back and the left arm is straight overhead. Repeat the movement.

This exercise will also expand the muscles at the outer edge of your shoulders, build up the forearms, and firm the muscles on the underside of your shoulder blades — a jackpot of benefits. Another bonus of this exercise is that it helps improve your posture. The movement conditions your muscles to hold your shoulders back without conscious thought during the day.

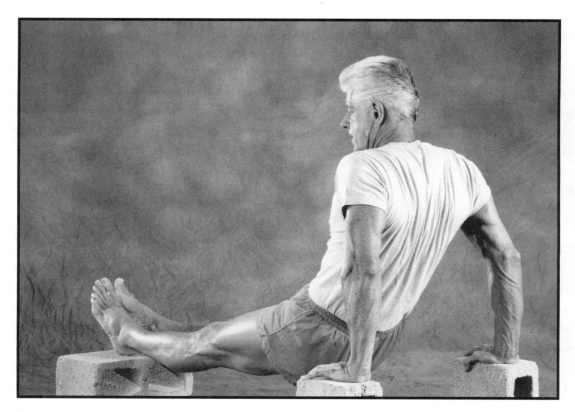

Reverse Dip

Reverse Dip

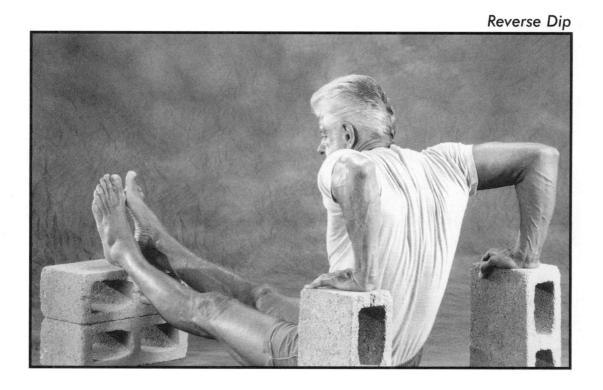

Reverse Dip

This is one of the oldest and most effective ways to remove flab from your upper chest, and to build your triceps and shoulders.

Version 1: Place two straight-back chairs or bricks face to face and slightly more than shoulder width apart. Place the palms of your hands on the chairs (or bricks, and extend your feet in front of you, keeping them straight throughout the exercise. Lower yourself until your buttocks are only a few inches above the floor,then push up to arms length.

Version 2: You can make the Reverse Dip more effective by using a low footstool for your feet, but you need to be in shape. Don't elevate your feet on a third chair — this creates balance problems that can result in severe muscle strain.

Forearm Pull

While standing, hold both ends of a towel in your left hand and grasp the loop of the towel in your right hand, palm down. Pull upward with your right hand while resisting with your left. Next pull downward with your left hand, resisting with your right. Then work the other side. This tones the forearms, improving your appearance in short sleeved shirts and blouses, and, believe it or not, giving you a better hand-shake.

Forearm Pull

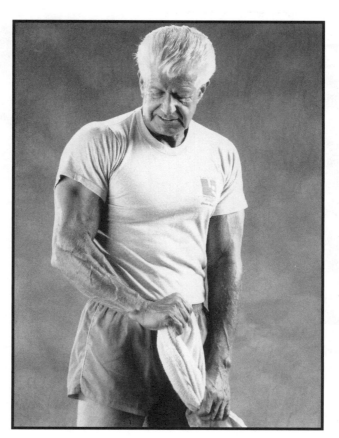

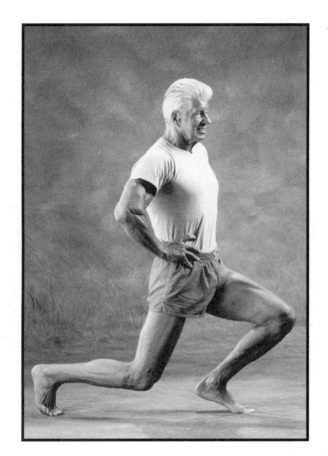

Thigh Lunge

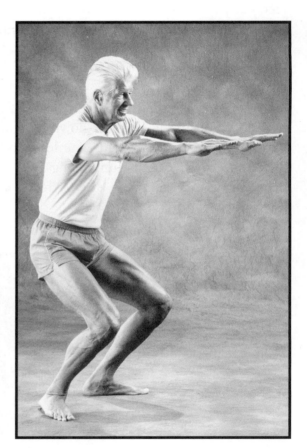

Half Knee Bend

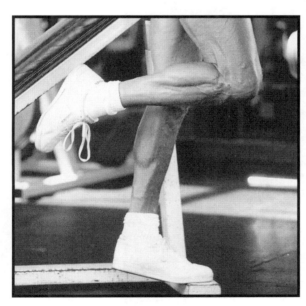

One-Legged Lunge

Thigh Lunge

Start with your hands on your hips and feet together. Take a long stride with your left foot, keeping the right leg extended behind you and your upper body perfectly erect. At full stretch your right knee will be just an inch or two off the floor. Warning: Do not exceed a 90 degree angle or you'll risk knee strain. Return to starting position. Now take a long stride with your right foot and touch your left knee to the floor. This exercise will help reduce the fatty tissue around your hips and thighs. It also conditions the quadriceps and, to a lesser degree, the hamstrings.

Half Knee Bend

We'll only hit the halfway point on the famous Knee Bend exercise because it's a real knee-popper unless you were born with exceptionally limber joints. A full Knee Bend risks the danger of torn knee cartilage, but the half measure will still give your thigh and calf muscles a good work-out.

Stand with your feet about 8 inches apart. Hold your arms straight in front of you at shoulder level for balance. Keeping your upper body erect, lower your hips to chair seat level or higher, then return to the upright position. As you straighten your legs, concentrate on using the muscles in your calves. Avoid doing too many of these if you're a beginner. Any knee bend exercise is deceiving, because you can typically accomplish several of them on the first effort, but may in fact be overtraining, which will result in severe soreness. Try holding a small telephone book for better balance. This exercise will help you build great legs.

Reverse Half Knee Bend

This is similar in concept to the Half Knee Bend, only you start below chair seat level and raise your torso halfway up, then back down. This is an effective exercise for those who want firm thighs, but be careful, this is for the advanced student.

One-Legged Calf Raise

While standing, place your left foot behind your right leg and brace yourself, then push yourself up and down to work the right calf muscles. Next, switch positions with your right foot behind your left leg and work the left calf muscles. If you really want to bring out those calf muscles, stand on a medium-sized telephone book and, balancing on the ball of your foot, lower yourself as slowly as you can. This exercise will help build a beautiful, well defined calf muscle.

• Five minutes of light aerobics (preferably walking or jogging in place)
• One stretching exercise for each muscle group (see chapter three)

Shoulders and Lats

• Shoulder Press
• Shoulder Swing
• Tug-Away (lats)

Chest and Back

• Push-Up
• Chair Dip (version 1, 2, or 3 depending on your ability)
• Pectoral Push

Biceps

• Concentration Towel Curl
• Muscle Curl
• Biceps Flex

Triceps

• Triceps Flex
• Triceps Press
• Reverse Dip (version 1 or 2 depending on your ability)

Forearm

• Forearm Pull

Legs

- Thigh Lunge
- Half Knee Bend
- Reverse Half Knee Bend
- One-Legged Calf Raises

Abdominal Exercises

- See Chapter Eight

Aerobics

- 15 to 30 minutes

Cool-Down

- Five minutes of light aerobics
- A few of your favorite stretches

Routine

Begin by performing 6 to 8 repetitions of each exercise, one time for the first week, twice for the second week. If you find this insufficient to give your muscles a good workout, add a couple more repetitions per exercise. I suggest doing the minimum number of repetitions during the first week, simply because your untrained muscles will be unaccustomed to exercise and are going to get sore. After a few weeks, you should be able to work up to 3 sets of 12 repetitions of each exercise, 3 times per week. Be sure to use good form on all exercises.

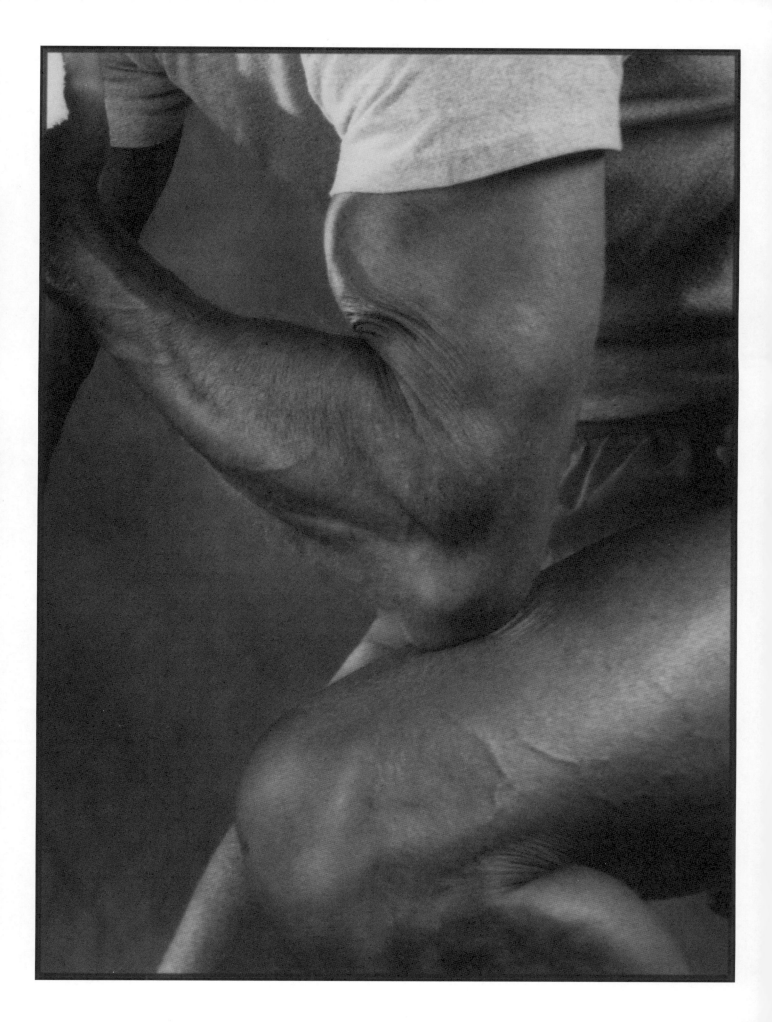

Tenets for Preventing Injuries

Before we go any further into the more intensive aerobic and weight training programs in the latter part of this book, I'd like to pause a moment to address what is probably your biggest concern about beginning any fitness regimen: the risk of injury. Somehow people have the idea that exercise has to hurt before it can help. This is not only inconsistent with all my research, but it's downright dangerous, especially for men and women in their thirties, forties, and beyond. The "no pain, no gain" philosophy can damage your muscles, break your spirit, and keep you from obtaining your fitness goals.

One reason I'm in good health is because in all my years of training, I've never once sustained an injury. What's my secret? I've always been in exceptional condition, thus eliminating any chance of injury from inactivity, I've never punished my body to the point of damaging the muscles or joints, and I've always known how to properly execute an exercise.

These are the tenets to preventing injuries. You need to be able to read your body and to know the difference between pain and harm. Too many people don't know their limits. Beginners, especially, start out with good intentions but often overtrain and damage their bodies. I've counseled and studied professional athletes, bodybuilders, and newcomers to the fitness world, and I've learned that you can't always predict what's going to happen, but you can decrease the odds of an injury through flexibility and strength training.

Chapter 6

I've called upon the foremost expert in the field of sports medicine, Dr. Leroy Perry, to provide answers to many of the mysteries surrounding fitness injuries and back pain. A writer, inventor, and practicing chiropractor to Hollywood stars, professionals, and Olympic athletes for more than three decades, he is sought after around the world as a consultant and lecturer.

Dr. Perry and I agree that the older we get, the more aches and pains we seem to have — a sore muscle here, a twinge there. Once discomfort evolves from subtle to prolonged and frequent, you've got a problem. Most older adults suffer from the usual pain, including backaches, headaches, and aches from old injuries. However, pain will likely strike a sedentary person before a physically fit one.

A certain number of aches and pains should be expected when you first start to exercise. Many of these will be caused by expanding muscles and shrinking fat. After a while, however, your strength will gradually improve and the constant throbbing in your body will lessen. Exercise may even help relieve certain kinds of chronic pain, but check with your doctor. Obviously, you shouldn't start a heavy weight-lifting program with a bad back.

Here are a few of the more common aches and pains that you may encounter during your training:

Muscle Pain and Soreness

If you're lifting weights, expect to experience some soreness in your muscles, but not to the point of excruciating pain. Most of the pain will be caused by microscopic tears to your muscle cells. These tears cause inflammation and swelling, but don't be alarmed — it's completely natural. That's actually how the muscle gets built up. But make sure you properly warm up before exercising and cool down after exercising. If you don't, the result could be serious damage to your muscles and joints. The more flexible you are, the better your ability to do more activity with less stress. You should also learn the correct form of each exercise and increase your intensity level gradually and over time. Don't try to "out-muscle" the person next to you.

If you're into walking, running, or some other aerobic activity, pace yourself. Shin splints — injury to and inflammation of the tibial muscles, usually caused by running on a hard surface — could set your training schedule back by weeks. Too many runners get carried away and run too fast, too hard, too soon. Enough is good, more than enough isn't. Increase your distance no more than 10 percent every week, because this allows your body to gradually absorb the added stress.

Also, avoid overloading the muscles, nerves, and bones, particularly your tendons. Avoid repeating a specific motion like a golf swing or a tennis player's serve, as these can cause tendonitis. If you do suffer from this problem, it could be your technique, in which case you should consult a specialist about reconditioning the affected muscle groups.

Stiff, Achy Joints

Joints are two or more bones held together by a variety of tissues, including tendons, ligaments, and muscles. They give you flexibility and motion, and provide a certain amount of support. As we get older, the joints and bones become more brittle, which increases our chances for fractures — especially of the hips. Other areas that may be affected by your exercise program are your back, knees, ankles, and shoulders. Additionally, worn cartilage and a lack of fluids in your joints may cause stiffness and make you less flexible.

Exercise and weight training can actually alleviate some of these problems, because they increase the calcium content of your bones. Naturally, the stronger the bones, the more demand you can place on your body. Exercise can also help if you have arthritis (inflammation of the joints). Remember, the best way to avoid injuries to your joints is to thoroughly warm up and cool down, and, since a lack of flexibility can lead to chronic aches, make sure you also stretch properly. If you do feel sore after your workout, you may want to consider taking a hot bath, a sauna or using a heating pad.

Feet and Ankle Damage

If your feet or ankles ache during or after aerobic activity, the problem could lie with your shoes. Some of the more common injuries to the feet include calluses and corns, which are caused by friction between foot and shoe. A burning sensation or shooting pain in the feet and legs can also result from wearing shoes that don't fit. To keep pain at a minimum, wear properly fitted shoes and stretch out your calf muscles. The best type of shoes have a good, solid heel cup, good support for the arch, and a big sole that absorbs shock. Spend the extra money for a good shoe that fits well and you won't regret it in the long run.

If you plan to make running regularly the cardiovascular component of your lifelong fitness program, you may want to consider wearing different running shoes — preferably two different brands — on alternate days. According to a recent report in Physician and Sports Medicine, this can reduce your risk of shin splints and other injuries because your feet and legs won't be subjected to the same stresses on every run. Another important consideration is to make sure you don't run in worn out shoes that have lost most of their shock absorbing capacity, thus subjecting your joints to additional stress.

Also, try to run on a well padded lawn or a soft dirt track. Running on asphalt or cement puts tremendous stress on your entire frame but is particularly bad for your feet, ankles, knees, and back. Shin splints are the result of running with your weight shifted too far forward, while Achilles tendonitis is caused by running with your weight too far back and striking your heel. Try not to overtrain, which tends to do more harm than good, and change your routine occasionally. Increase and decrease your intensity levels every other week. Allow yourself sufficient time to rest so that your body can repair itself.

Your ankles are supported by ligaments only. The ligaments running down the front and back of your ankles are relatively weak, while the ones running along the sides are strong and thick. Most of you have probably experienced a sprained ankle or tears of the ligaments at some time in your life — a simple fall or misstep can set your training schedule back by weeks. The key to avoiding injuries in this area is to increase the flexibility and strength of the ankle ligaments through simple calf stretches and raises. These exercises help you maintain full range of motion in your ankles.

Headaches and Backaches

Headaches, neck and back pain, the daily tensions that slow you down and make you feel prematurely old are all typically the result of back problems and poor posture. Obviously, there may be other, more serious reasons for these conditions, but, in most cases, I'm willing to bet those aches and pains stem from the problems I've just outlined. Even people who are in exceptional condition feel, at some period during their lives, a sense of discomfort in their backs. A lot of people throw their backs out just bending over to pick up a towel. If you've never had a back problem, consider yourself lucky. Roughly 90 percent of all Americans will suffer at least one backache. What causes all those backs to ache?

Lack of physical activity is a strong possibility. "Researchers have found a strong correlation between weak stomach muscles and chronic back pain," says Dr. Perry. He adds that "persistent pain may be helped with simple and slow concentrated exercises focused on hitting the abdominal muscles." This position was reinforced by a study at the University of Miami that found strong evidence that exercise can relieve certain kinds of back pain.

As mentioned, however, chronic pain may stem from a congenital defect of which you aren't aware, which is why you should always consult a doctor first. Maybe you have a vertebra that didn't form properly, or structural instabilities that won't go away. Here are a few danger signs and symptoms of possible back problems that should be checked by your physician, a sports medicine specialist, or an orthopedic surgeon:

- Pain that goes from your back all the way down your leg toward your foot, or down your arm toward your hand
- Back pain that continues for more than two weeks
- Numbness in your leg, foot, arm or hand
- Pain in your back that keeps you from sleeping

Barring any existing problems dating from birth, exercise and proper stretching, in conjunction with abdominal exercises, will help most backaches. Dr. Perry and I agree that the greatest majority of back problems are the result of a back that's too strong in comparison to the abdominal muscles. As you age, the abdominal muscles naturally get weaker and the lower back gets tighter, causing the abdomen — which is actually the front of your back — to protrude. According to Dr. Perry, the great majority of older Americans have weak stomach muscles. A pot belly is almost guaranteed to adversely affect your posture and put added stress on your lower back. Therefore, the important factors for correcting back problems are flexibility, balance, endurance, and strength in the abdominal area.

Researchers at the University of Miami placed a number of people with serious back problems on an exercise program that included stretching and calisthenics. After only two weeks, most of the sufferers had succeeded in easing their pain. Increasingly, researchers are realizing that the strength and flexibility of your back, stomach, and hip muscles will almost certainly bring relief. Here are a few basic suggestions to help ward off back problems:

- Keep your abdominal muscles strong to help compensate for an unstable back.
- Improve your posture by learning to keep your chest up and head high, neck straight, hips forward, stomach firm, and buttocks relaxed.
- Sleep on a firm mattress, preferably on your side, or with a pillow under your neck.
- Learn to lift objects properly: Bend at the knees, keeping your back straight and using only your leg muscles.
- Supplement your Calcium intake, up to 3000 mg daily.

The following exercises, designed by Dr. Perry and myself, will strengthen your back and stomach muscles, improve your posture, help alleviate the pressure on your spine caused by gravity, and generally make you feel and look 10 years younger. This program has been proven to be effective in relieving pain and restoring function and mobility for many muscle and joint problems.

These exercises are a combination of ancient and modern methods, drawing both on Dr. Perry's knowledge of contemporary chiropractic sports science, and on my experience as a health and fitness consultant. Using these stretching exercises before you train will reduce the chance of injury to muscles, tendons, and ligaments, and doing them after you train will help keep you limber and help prepare your body for the next day. Use common sense. Don't try to stretch too fast and too soon, or you will do serious damage to your body. If your doctor has given you permission to undertake an exercise program, but you're still concerned about hurting your back, I recommend you master these stretches before proceeding any further with the program.

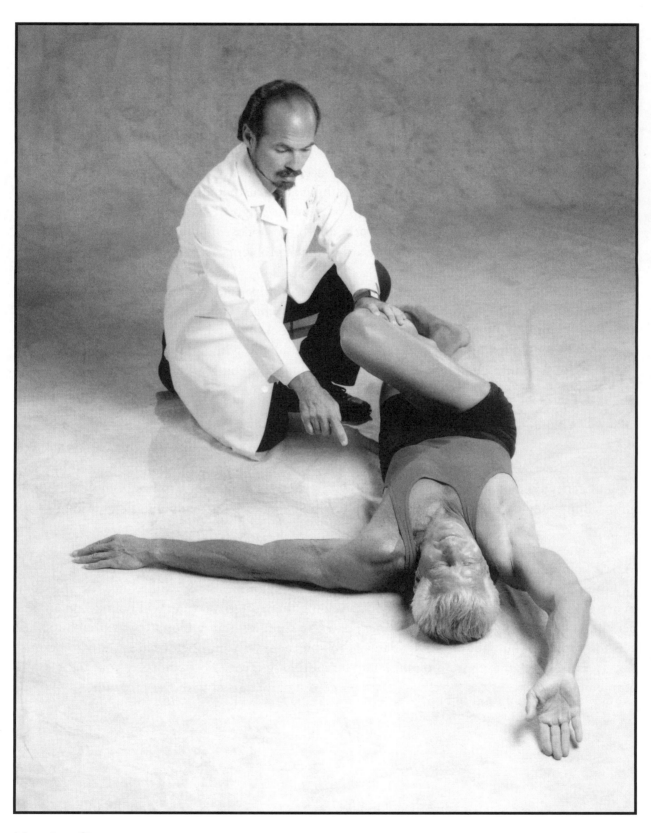

Morning Star

Morning Star

Lie on your back with your right arm stretched overhead, pointing north, and your left arm extended at a 90 degree angle, pointing east. Swing your right leg up and over your left leg, and try to touch your right knee to the ground. Breathe and relax. Hold for several seconds. You should feel a stretch in your lower and upper back, your hamstrings, and your gluteus muscles (the large muscles of the buttocks). Stretch the other side, this time with your left arm overhead, and your right arm at a 90 degree angle. If you can't bring your knee to the floor on the opposite side of your leg, don't fret. Eventually you'll be limber enough to hold this position for up to five full seconds.

Leg and Torso Stretch

Lie on your stomach with your hands at your sides, palms up. First raise the right leg as high as you can without discomfort. Try not to bend your leg at the knee. Hold it briefly at the peak of the raise, then lower. Next, lift your left leg the same way. Move your head up and back as far as you can and lift your torso. You probably won't be able to hold your torso at the peak of the raise for more than an instant.

Crunch #1

Lie on your back, knees bent, feet flat on the floor. With your hands behind your head, tighten your gluteus and abdominal muscles by slowly pulling your head forward until you feel a slight stretch in the lower back. Concentrate on curling your abdominal muscles by tucking your pubic bone up toward your navel. This particular exercise is easier on the spine than a normal sit-up, and it concentrates on developing your lower abdominal muscles.

Crunch #2

While still on your back, feet flat on the floor, place a pillow between your upper thighs and squeeze. Fold your arms across your chest, and slowly raise your head enough to curl your chin into your chest and hold. Your shoulder blades should remain on the floor even at the highest point of the curl. Return to starting position. Gradually increase your "hold" to several seconds.

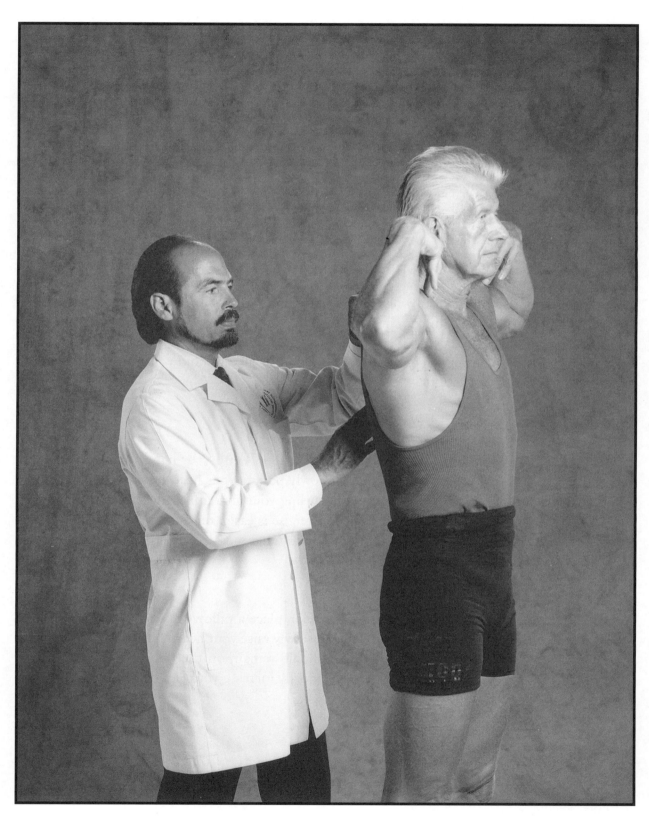

Reverse Shoulder Shrugs #2

Pelvic Tilt

Stand facing a wall and place a pillow between your upper thighs. With your arms overhead, palms against the wall, and feet flat, lean your body into the wall at a 45 degree angle. Squeeze the pillow with your upper and lower abdominal muscles and upper thigh muscles, and curl and tuck your pubic bone into your navel. Do not tighten your buttocks or back. Hold for several seconds, relax. This exercise will help flatten your stomach, decrease sway, and aid in realigning your lower back. It can also make a significant contribution to the improvement of your posture.

Reverse Shoulder Shrugs #1

Stand in front of a mirror, arms at your sides. With your chest fully expanded, shrug your shoulders up toward your ears, then back, then down — to improve flexibility in your upper back and to realign your spine, neck, and head. Try to make your shoulder blades touch. Hold for several seconds, then relax. This exercise will strengthen your shoulders to help you carry your head and neck more gracefully.

Reverse Shoulder Shrugs #2

Same exercise as before, only bend your arms at the elbows, and touch your shoulders with your hands. Complete the exercise by rolling your shoulders up toward your ears, back, and then down. Hold for several seconds, then return to original position.

Backward Neck Press

Place both hands on the back of your head. Apply resistance to the back of your head while steadily pressing backward with your head and neck. This exercise helps you tone and strengthen the back of your neck, forcing your head and neck to align with your spine. The more your head protrudes forward, the greater the stress on your neck and the more your spinal cord is stretched. This can aggravate lower-back problems and cause headaches, according to Dr. Perry.

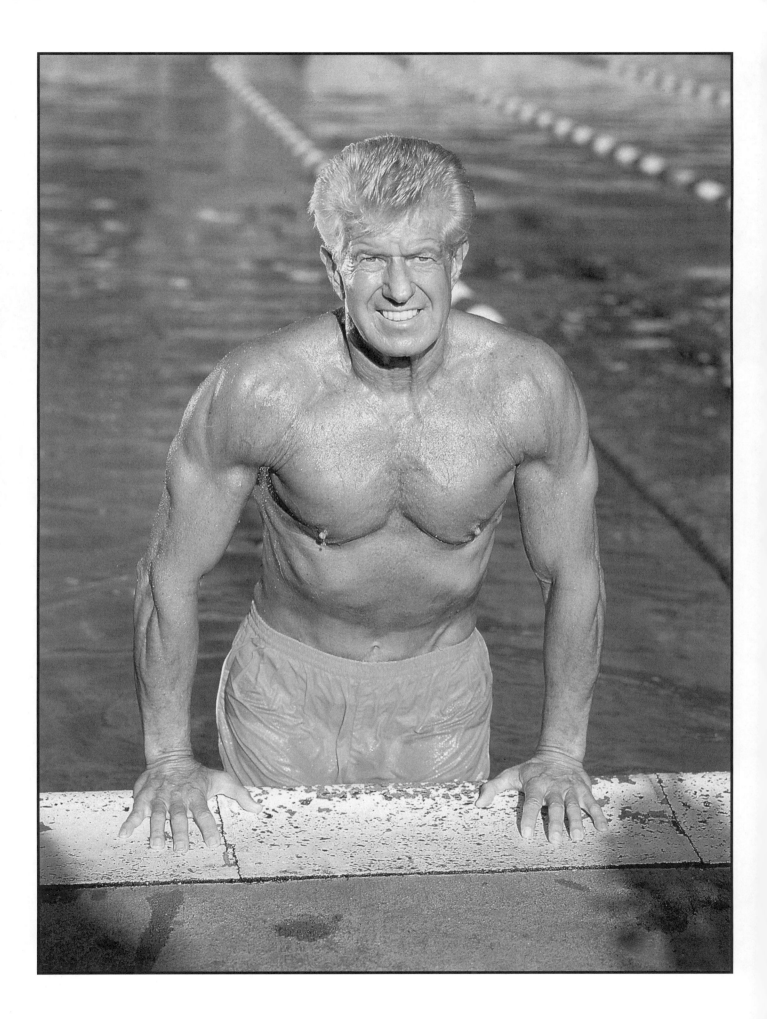

Stamina and Endurance

Now that you've familiarized yourself with my Isotension Program, and have learned basic stretches that will increase your flexibility and prevent injuries, it's time to tackle the next component of any truly effective exercise regimen: cardiovascular conditioning. It's no longer just science fiction. Based on current theories being passed around the scientific community, including pioneering work in the study of what controls aging, aerobic activities such as walking, jogging, swimming, and cycling can increase your life expectancy. The mere notion that we can do something today about living longer tomorrow should have you excited about exercise in general and cardiovascular conditioning in particular. Perhaps the most compelling bit of evidence that exercise extends your life came several years ago from a project known as the Harvard Alumni Study. Researchers tracked the life-styles of more than 16,000 Harvard graduates, ages 35 to 74. The results showed positive evidence that men who regularly exercise or walk long distances can expect to add one to two years to their lives by the time they reach 80. Research also confirms that your heart and lungs begin to decline with age. As a result, your metabolism and the oxygen that's delivered to your muscles declines, as well. But the effects of aging are no longer considered irreversible. Several studies, including the one conducted at Tufts University, have shown that strong muscles, a low-fat diet, and an increase in your oxygen utilization can all but guarantee you better health and longer life.

The type of aerobic activity you do doesn't seem to matter, as long as you breathe oxygen into your body about as fast as you use it. It may surprise you to learn that there is nothing exotic or new about any of the aerobic activities I recommend in my program. I've had the opportunity to research an almost unlimited supply of the most priceless commodity in the health and fitness industry — the human body. Although today's training equipment is sophisticated and efficient, I've come to realize that the best way to live longer — and on your own terms — is through the basic exercises that have been around since, well, mankind.

Most aerobic activities are incredibly simple, and amazingly effective. Certainly, stair-climbing machines, treadmills, and stationary bikes are great if they're available, but you don't need to be a member of a health club to get a decent workout. One of the reasons I'm so healthy at 80 is because every day for the last 50 years I've either walked, jogged, or cycled. Some activities produce quicker results than others, but as long as you're huffing and puffing, and as long as you've got the proper motivation, my program will work. Remember, successful aerobic activity is measured in a heightened heart rate, not in how much you sweat.

What Specifically Will Aerobics Do for You?

- Increase the efficiency of your lungs, conditioning them to process more oxygen with less effort.
- Increase the strength of your heart and lower your heart rate, so that it will pump more blood, reducing your chances of a stroke or heart attack. (Generally, people with a resting heart rate in the 40-beats-per-minute range are in exceptional condition; those with a resting heart rate in the 60s are in good condition; those with a resting heart rate in the 80s are in poor condition.)
- Increase the size of your blood vessels, often reducing your blood pressure sure so that the vessels can carry blood and energy producing oxygen to the body tissues, giving you more stamina, endurance, and energy.
- Raise metabolism to a rate that burns stored fat, helping to change your fat weight into lean-muscle weight.
- Increase your oxygen consumption and improve the overall condition of your body (you can do more work with less effort).
- Change your whole outlook on life because you'll learn to relax, develop a better self-image, and be better equipped to handle the stresses of everyday living.
- Give you more stamina, endurance and energy.

Learn to Walk Before You Run

In order to get a complete aerobic workout that will yield the most benefits, the exercise needs to be vigorous enough so that you're within 50 percent to 85 percent of your maximum heart rate, according to the American College of Sports Medicine (ACSM). Your maximum heart rate is roughly 200 minus your age. A 40-year-old woman, for example, would have a maximum heart rate of 160 beats per minute. If she were interested in staying within 60 percent of that target range, she would multiply 160 by 60 percent for 96 beats per minute.

To produce a sustained heart rate while exercising, you need to learn how to take your pulse. This may seem elementary to some, but it's an important component of your aerobic program. Place the index and middle fingers of your right hand over your left wrist. Feel around for your pulse. Did you find it? Count the beats for 10 seconds and multiply by 6.

Monitoring your heart rate during exercise helps you measure the effectiveness of your workout. If you're working out above your target heart range, you may be working too hard, in which case you should lower your intensity. If you're below your target heart range, you may want to increase the intensity. For those of you interested simply in maintaining your health and maximizing the fat-burning effects of aerobic activity, an intensity level of 60 percent to 75 percent is ideal. If you're a beginner you should exercise at the lower end of your target heart range until you feel comfortable with stepping up your exercise intensity. If you're in great shape, use the formula of 200 minus your age for your target heart range.

Your aerobic schedule should be kept at 20 to 60 minutes in length, 3 times per week. As your condition improves, you can work up to 5 times per week, although as aerobic impact activities increase, so does the chance of injury unless you're conscientious. The ACSM recommends that you participate in aerobic exercise — on alternate days during the initial conditioning stages.

Surprisingly, your aerobic exercise doesn't have to be as strenuous as you may assume. A study at the Cooper Institute for Aerobics Research found that a 12 minute-per-mile walk improves your cardiovascular fitness just as well as a 9 minute-per-mile jog. A second study at the same institute reported that a person can still lose weight at a 20 minute-per-mile pace. Researchers further noted that all of the strollers increased the levels of their "good" cholesterol, and that those walkers who got up to 60 percent of their maximum oxygen consumption (amount of oxygen your body uses during a workout) lowered their risk of heart disease by 18 percent.

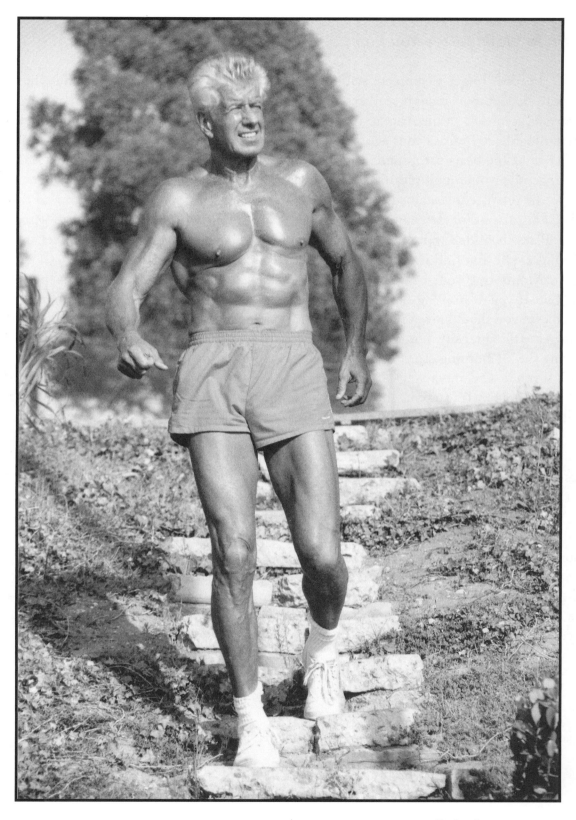

Learn to walk before you run

Despite the obvious benefits of cardiovascular exercise, your muscles and tendons will need time to adjust to the new and increased stresses. For the over 30 crowd, leg and back muscles, especially, may become extremely sore. Be sure to spend 5 to 8 minutes warming up prior to participating in any aerobic activity. Some stretching, slow jogging, walking, or stationary running are good. If you're running or walking long distances, you may prefer to incorporate the warm-up into the early minutes of your routine. When you're finished with your aerobic activity, spend another 5 to 8 minutes warming down by walking or jogging around the block. After vigorous exercise involving primarily the legs, most of the blood is pooled in the legs. Be aware that it takes a few minutes for this blood to get back into general circulation.

Walking

Walking is the safest and easiest form of exercise known to mankind, and probably the most neglected. Walking helps to reduce the heartbeat and lower the blood pressure; increase metabolism, stamina, and energy levels; and improve circulation. It's also a great fat burner. One study reported in the journal of the American Medical Association found that walking improves a person's blood cholesterol balance. A second study discovered a relationship between walking and stronger bones. Hippocrates, the great Greek patron of medicine, prescribed walking as a cure-all for medical and mental problems. He said you have two doctors — your right leg and your left leg — and whenever your body and your mind are out of sync you need to just call on your two doctors and invariably you shall be healed.

Cardiovascular and respiratory functions begin to decline with age. If you don't exercise, the slide accelerates rapidly. The heart, too, begins to function less efficiently. If you want to improve your overall health, increase endurance, and take your shot at living a longer, more satisfactory life — start walking today.

Happily, more and more people are becoming aware of walking's benefits. More than 70 million Americans report that they walk for at least part of their weekly exercise routine because it's easy and virtually injury-free, and makes so few demands on the body. Anyone can do it. It's a natural exercise that doesn't require a great deal of strength. Older people, even children, have decided to walk as their exercise. So should you. But you can't be a schlepper. You've got to put out the effort. Window-shopping speed is fine, for a while. But you must eventually elevate your heart rate or it doesn't do your cardiovascular system much good. I try to make walking a daily venture by constantly finding new and exciting paths, which alleviates boredom.

Start your conditioning by jogging in place. Push upward from your toes to work your calf muscles, and lift your knees about waist-high. The key is to keep your heart pumping. Try to keep your arms limber, your neck muscles relaxed. This is great warm-up and cool-down exercise. Begin by limiting yourself to one or two minutes in the morning and evening, especially if you've been sedentary all your life. Increase gradually until you can comfortably do 5 minutes at least 3 times a week.

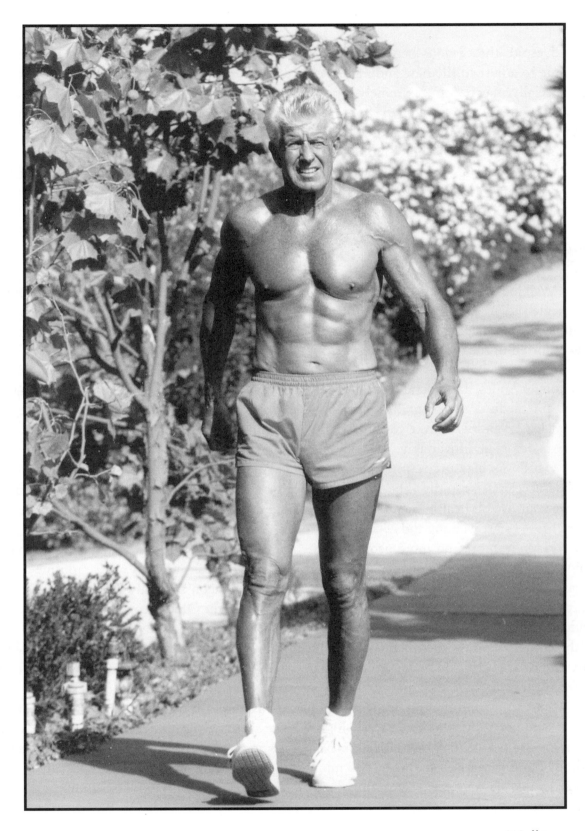

Walking

Although it seems obvious, sometimes we need to be reminded that walking should start with your feet positioned properly. This means your lead foot should land with your weight slightly in front of the heel, allowing the foot to roll through the arch and push off with your toes. The more efficient your foot movement, the better the workout for your legs. Start by walking around the block. Keep your chest high, your abdomen in, and your body relaxed.

To get an "aerobic" effect from walking, you either must cover a long distance or walk fairly fast. Walking 3 miles in 45 minutes provides more cardiovascular benefit than running 1 mile in under 6 minutes — and there's less risk of injury. The anaerobic effect (meaning without oxygen) you get from sprinting is good only if you're a serious athlete. Stick to the exercises that yield an "aerobic" effect. And remember to stay within your target heart range. Monitor your pulse every 10 minutes. Increase your intensity if you're not working hard enough, and decrease it if you're working too hard.

Your walk should be moderately paced and relaxed. If you've been inactive for a while, start by walking slowly for short distances, and gradually work up to a faster pace and longer distances. But don't push yourself too hard. For injury-free walking, use Dr. Perry's advice for proper technique: Lean forward slightly, push off with your rear foot, and keep your pubic bone tucked up and your upper body properly aligned.

Walking correctly helps you use the muscles of your body more efficiently. It also helps improve coordination and balance. The primary benefit is that it allows your muscles to do what they're supposed to do, which is pump oxygen and blood throughout your body. But keep it simple. The best way to walk is by doing what comes naturally.
The following tips should help you increase your distance and enjoyment:

- Gentle stretching before you walk will help prevent soreness and injury.
- Walk on a soft surface (a track or dirt), and on level ground.
- If you experience pain, stop and rest, then resume.
- Try to walk at least 4 times a week.

If the weather is bad, try walking in a mall or some other indoor space, or jog in place in your home. Don't forget to cool down after you exercise. It's important because your muscles shorten slightly as a result of strenuous exercise, and this can cause soreness. By going through a cool-down routine you prep the muscles for the next day's workout. One of the best ways to cool down is to continue walking but at a slower than normal pace, while slightly increasing your overall range of motion. This also helps increase flexibility.

Jogging

Both walking and jogging are excellent exercises. Both are also great ways to reduce the daily tensions in your life, and result in better general health habits. Don't feel you're confined to a particular route, distance, or level of intensity once you've established an exercise routine. It's possible to control the degree of exertion by varying the distance, speed of running, and amount of walking. I happen to do both, depending on my mood. I used to jog for 12 minutes. Then it was for 15 minutes. These days, I jog for 20 to 30 minutes, 4 to 5 times a week depending on my schedule.

You should try to enjoy your run — don't make it a chore or you're less likely to stick with it. My recommendation is that you combine walking and jogging, gradually increasing your pace and distance. Take a day off between jogging days. Once your condition improves, you can go 4 to 5 times a week.

When walking, you naturally start slowly, gradually increasing the distance and the pace. This puts less stress on the heart, lungs, and muscles. When walking and jogging, you increase or decrease your pace and style according to your ability. if you're in good physical condition, you can do more jogging. If you're in poor shape,you can do more walking. The goal is to train yourself to the point where you can mostly jog, or achieve a heart rate consistently in your target zone. I know of a 70 year old woman in Santa Monica, California, who started this routine four years ago, and today she's running marathons. At the very least, it will leave you more vital and alive.

Unlike anaerobic activities such as weight lifting, isotonic exercises, and calisthenics, jogging improves your heart, lungs, and circulatory system. This makes jogging and other cardiovascular activities imperative for anyone over 30. After all, bulging biceps may boost your ego and impress your friends, but a healthy heart and lungs will extend your life.

Here are some other benefits of a good cardiovascular program:

- It makes you feel and look younger.
- It helps you lose weight by burning fat.
- It builds endurance, energy, and confidence.
- It gives you a smaller waistline.

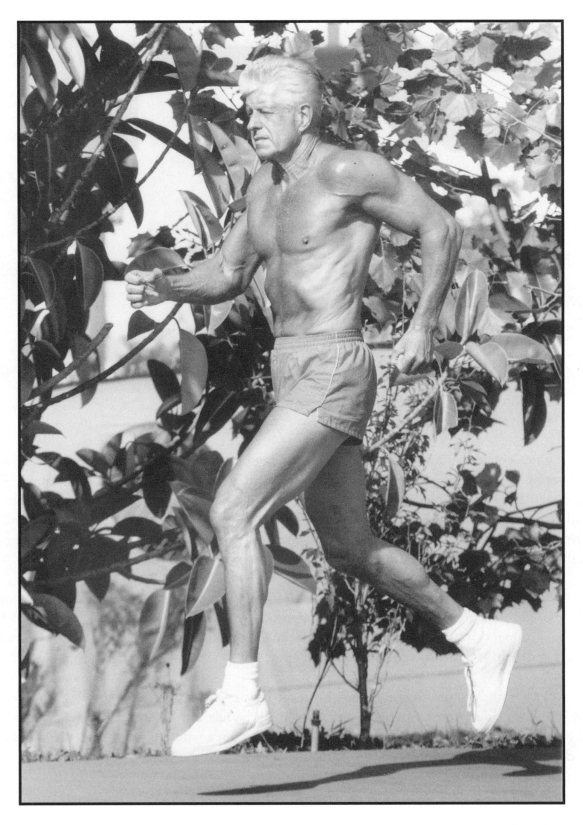

Jogging

Dr. Leroy Perry has worked with hundreds of professional and Olympic athletes, ever since he became the first chiropractor to serve as an official Olympic team doctor. He advises that you do the following when jogging:

DO

- Plant your foot at a point 3/4 inches forward of your heel
- Push off with the ball and toes of your back foot.
- Lean your body 10 to 20 degrees forward.
- Swing your arms in a relaxed manner, like a free pendulum.
- Look at the horizon, not the ground.
- Relax your hands and jaw.

DON'T

- Run with short, choppy strides.
- Cross your feet in front of each other.
- Swing your arms around your body.
- Tighten your hands or clench your jaw.
- Let your body dehydrate.

Once you're comfortable enough with walking or jogging to try a more advanced routine, buy a set of hand weights, although make sure you're in great shape before you do. Many walkers and joggers have added hand weights to their program to attain a higher level of fitness. It builds stamina and strength, and it's a great complement to your training program. A study at the University of Pittsburgh's Human Energy Research Lab found that people who pumped 2 pound weights while jogging burned 120 more calories per half hour than those who didn't.

The theory behind walking with hand-held weights is that jogging or walking alone won't build muscles in the upper part of your body, especially your arms. You may have noticed how marathon runners always look extremely thin, lacking any real definition of their biceps or triceps. Using hand-held weights builds muscle in the upper torso.

Start with 2 pound weights. The proper technique is to begin by walking. Let the weights dangle by your sides. Your arms and shoulders should be relaxed. Begin pumping your hands up and down, as if you were doing biceps curls. It may take you a while to get your rhythm, but once you do, the awkwardness of the movement should do most of the work.

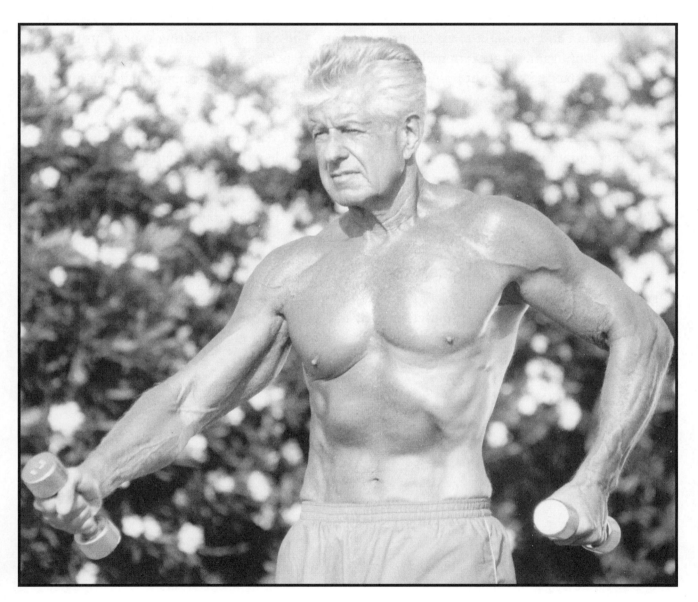

Walking with weights

A note of caution: Never wear ankle weights while walking or jogging. Some people, aware of the benefits of working with hand weights while running, have assumed this applies to ankle weights as well. This is not the case. The added weight adds strain to your knee and ankle joints as your legs flow through their full range of motion. That's like adding a weight to a swinging pendulum and forcing it to exceed its natural arc. The chances of injuring your joints or over straining your ligaments are extremely high. Since I'll be showing you how to strengthen your legs through resistance and weight training exercises, there's no reason to attempt to build leg muscles using ankle weights.

My aerobic schedule is 2 days in a row, and then 1 day off, or roughly 5 times per week. I'll either run an under 8 minute mile, jog 2 1/2 miles in less than 20 minutes, or ride the stationary bike for 20 minutes (100 — 120 RPM). If you have access to a stair-climbing machine, stationary bike, treadmill, or other cardiovascular exercise machine that will give you a good aerobic workout, by all means use them to your advantage. Varying your schedule and even your activities keeps you from "burning out" on one exercise.

Of course, no amount of walking, jogging, or any other aerobic activity will do you any good unless it's done at between 50 percent to 85 percent of your maximum heart rate, a pace that's fast enough to work your muscles, heart, and lungs. A realistic goal is 3 half-hour sessions every week. After only a few weeks you'll notice not only physical changes to your body, but also improvements to your mental state.

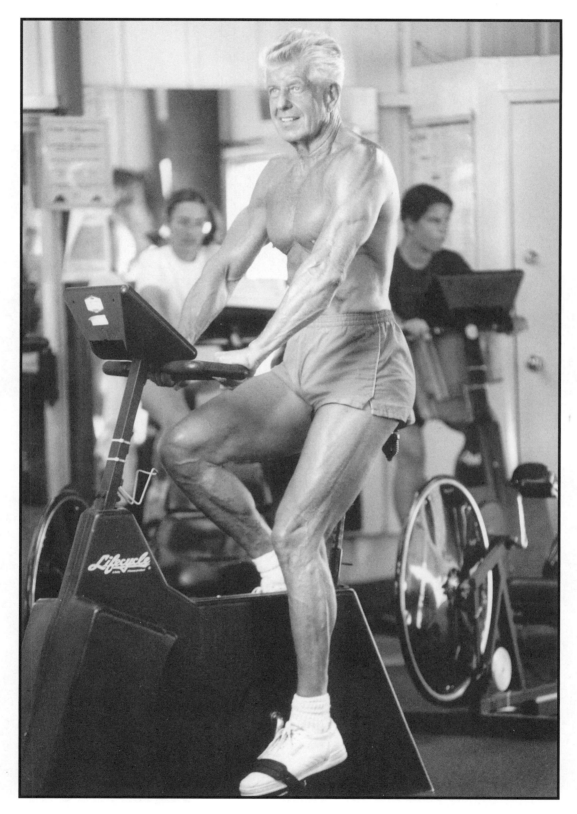

Stationary Bike

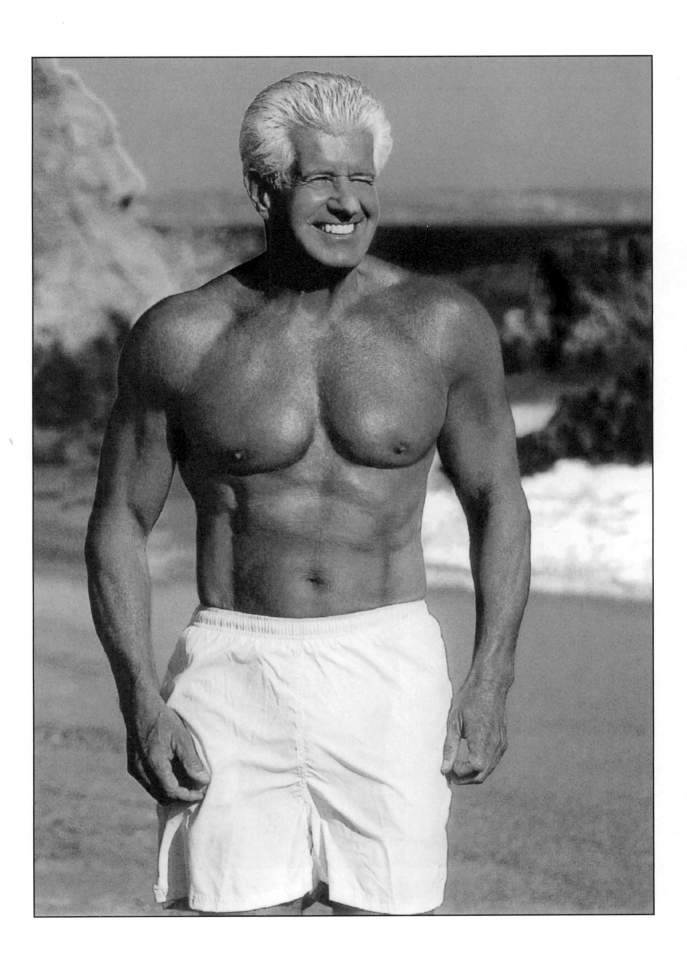

Phase Three: Strength Training and Muscle Building

One of the most exciting developments in the health and fitness field during the last decade has been the medical community's endorsement of weight training and strength conditioning as a way of staving off the effects of aging. Pumping iron does more than just produce bulging biceps and impressive triceps. According to the latest research, it can also increase your metabolic rate and burn body fat, and literally add years to your life.

According to a study at the University of Missouri — Columbia School of Medicine, men lose lean body mass gradually, starting at about age 41, while women lose lean body mass after menopause. The study tracked 564 men and 61 women over the age of 18 and reaffirmed that any decline in lean body mass wreaks havoc on your metabolism which, in turn, causes you to burn fewer calories and gain more weight. This vicious cycle, however, can be stopped by incorporating weight training into your exercise program, because weight training builds lean body mass.

According to a study conducted by the University of Maryland in conjunction with the Baltimore Veterans Administration Medical Center, a group of sedentary older men increased their strength by 38 percent and lean body mass by an average of 4 pounds after only 12 weeks of resistance training. A 2000 study published in the journal of the American Medical Association reported a 48 percent increase in mobility and a substantial increase in strength among 10 90-year-old subjects who had strength trained for only 8 weeks. What I find most interesting about these studies is they prove you don't have to work out with the intensity of a professional bodybuilder to reap the benefits of weight training.

Benefits of Weight Training and Bodybuilding

- Greater ability to burn fat, because of greater muscle mass and higher activity level
- Greater strength and mobility
- Stronger bones and joints
- Better coordination and control over one's muscles
- Lower risk of heart disease (thanks to a combined effort of weight training, diet, and cardiovascular training)
- Better attitude and improved mood (apparently because of better nervous system functioning and the release of endorphins, natural opiates in the brain that are released during or after strenuous exercise)
- Continued mobility and independence in old age
- Vastly improved self-image, thanks to a better-looking body
- Makes you more attractive
- Give you better posture, and a sense of well-being

Proper Weight and Intensities

Muscles are made up of fibers that are held together by elastic connective tissue. The fibers themselves are made up of cells. Weight training helps you preserve and build lean muscle mass by increasing the size of the cells. You can build muscle by lifting a weight up, and by putting it back down. Weight-lifting equipment is designed specifically to augment this process.

The barbell consists of a long bar with some sort of locking device at each end so that you can add or remove plates. Dumbbells are hand-held weights with similar plates and locking devices. Barbells, dumbbells (I'd suggest a 120 pound set if you're a beginner, a 210 pound set for the more advanced student), and a two-way bench for flat and incline positions, are the only tools you'll need to get started. An increase in strength can be achieved at home, using home-made or store bought weights, or at the gym. Many people seem to prefer the multifaceted machines that can work nearly every muscle group.

Whether you decide to work out at home or in a gym, you must find the appropriate weight for each exercise. I've noticed that most people use too much weight when they work out, which causes them to do the exercise incorrectly. My suggestion is that you work within 50 percent to 80 percent (depending on your condition) of your **maximum lifting weight** — the absolute heaviest weight you can lift on each exercise (if you can lift it a second time, it's too light). For example, if the most you can bench press one time is 140 pounds, you need to work out with between 70 and 120 pounds to stay within 50 percent to 80 percent of your target range. Be sure to use a weight that you can handle smoothly, with proper form and rhythm.

Don't be afraid to mix up your routine or devise your own. As long as you follow the basic program I've outlined, or a variation thereof, you'll be assured tremendous results. You may find yourself getting burned out on one routine, in which case you should revert to one of the others. Don't forget that the Isotension Program is great for those times you can't get to the gym. The most important element of any weight training program is simply to use a weight that works best for you.

If you're out of shape, or have a medical problem of any kind, first consult your physician for approval. The American College of Sports Medicine advises all middle-aged and older individuals to start any exercise program by visiting a doctor who can measure their aerobic and muscle condition. A high-intensity weight training program can increase your muscle strength, but it can also cause injuries. Always begin with a comfortable weight, especially if you're a beginner. Increase the weight slowly, over time, and never to the point of injuring your muscles or hurting yourself.

Before You Get Started

Here are some important considerations to keep in mind as you begin the Lifelong Fitness program of weight training:

- Do not hold your breath when lifting weights. Breathing is essential to a proper workout. Exhale as you push and inhale as you pull.
- Breathe through your mouth when exercising, and be sure to breathe from the lower abdomen.
- Lift slowly and avoid jerky, explosive movements. Form is everything. Exercise with rhythm.
- Make sure your training is suited to your personal objectives: Heavy lifting tends to build a strong, heavily muscled body, while lighter lifting tends to build a toned body.
- Give your muscles time to rest and rebuild. Give yourself a full 24 to 48 hours of rest between weight workouts — more is not always better.
- Proper execution of the exercise is key. Don't cheat.
- Always run through a series of warm-up exercises before you exercise, as well as a proper cool-down session afterward.

Building Strong Muscles

A well developed body is one of the nicest rewards of pursuing lifelong fitness. It not only gives you a more youthful appearance, but it frees you of the physical limitations that come about as the result of aging and inactivity. But in order to achieve good muscle tone and strength, you must work all the major muscle groups in your body. A well rounded weight-lifting program targets two key areas: Your upper body (chest, arms, shoulders, and back), your lower body (hips, buttocks, and legs), and your abdomen.

Here are descriptions of the various muscles you'll be exercising. Keep in mind that physical size is not always a good barometer of how well you're doing. The primary hallmarks of good muscular function are strength, endurance, and flexibility.

Shoulders. Your deltoids are the large triangular muscles that run along the upper part of the shoulder blades at the collarbone. This set of muscles typically doesn't get challenged very often, but they're important for maintaining that broad shouldered look and for good posture.

Back. Your latissimus dorsi travels upward along the spine and sideways to the shoulder. Your trapezius muscles are the large flat triangular muscles that form along each side of the back. Well developed back muscles give you that V-shape look that so many people try to achieve, and they also make your waist appear smaller.

Chest. The pectoralis is another muscle that typically doesn't get used much in day-to-day living. The two-headed muscle that runs along the front of the upper breastbone, it connects the walls of the chest to the bones of the upper arms and shoulders. Well developed chest muscles give you a firm, well-toned look and help you hold up those areas that gravity wants to pull down.

Biceps and Triceps. Your biceps are the two-headed flexor muscles on the front side of your upper arms. Your triceps are the three-headed extensor muscles that run along the back side of your upper arms and attach to your shoulder blades. Both muscle groups have a tendency to sag with age, particularly in women. Strong biceps and triceps, however, improve the overall strength and endurance of your upper body.

Legs. Our lower bodies are responsible for everyday movement, including walking and jogging. If we neglect the hips, buttocks, and legs, we limit our freedom to lead an active life. Your hamstring muscles are located on the back of the thighs, while your quadriceps are on the front. The calves are the fleshy part of your legs below the back of your knees that tie in with the Achilles tendons. All three help protect against extra stress on the knee and maintain muscular balance. Lower body strength improves overall mobility and stability.

Abdomen. Chapter Nine is devoted to detailed advice about developing and maintaining strong abdominal muscles.

The following weight-training programs are designed for use in a gym. If you have never worked out in a gym before, and are unfamiliar with the equipment I discuss, I suggest you ask a trainer in your gym to go through the purpose and proper procedure for each piece of gym equipment. I've outlined programs for various levels of fitness. If you're out of shape and overweight, or if you've never lifted a weight in your life, start with the Beginner's Weight-Training Program outlined below. If you're a weekend athlete or if you've been training somewhat regularly for at least three months, you should go with the Intermediate program. You should place yourself in the Advanced program only if 1) you've been training hard for at least six months and 2) you really want to concentrate on sculpting your body. Most of you should work up to, or stay with, the Intermediate level of training. To move from one level to the next, you should be able to do 3 sets of each exercise (8 to 15 reps) without any discomfort.

Beginner's Weight-Training Program

Warm-Up

- Five minutes of a light aerobic activity (walking or jogging in place)
- One stretching exercise for each muscle group (see Chapter Four)

Shoulders

- Upright Row (Barbell)
- Standing Shoulder Press (Barbell)
- Seated Shoulder Press (Dumbbells)
- Side Laterals (Dumbbells)

Back

- Lat Pull Downs
- Rowing (Dumbbells)

Chest

- Bench Press (Barbell)
- Flyes (Dumbbells)
- Incline Chest Press (Dumbbells)
- Pullover (Barbell)

Triceps

- Triceps Extension (Dumbbells)
- Triceps Extension (Barbell)
- Kick Back (Dumbbells)

Biceps

- Barbell Curl
- Seated Dumbbell Curl
- Concentrated Dumbbell Curl

Legs

- Half-Squats
- Leg Extension
- Leg Curl
- Two-Legged Calf Raise

Abdominals

- See Chapter Eight

Aerobics

- 20 to 45 minutes at 55 percent to 75 percent of your maximum heart rate, 3 to 4 days per week

Cool-Down

- Five minutes of a light aerobic activity

Routine

If you're a beginner, I recommend that you begin slowly during the first several weeks. Lift weights in a slow, controlled manner, over the course of several seconds. Instead of performing the usual 3 sets of 10 to 12 repetitions, start by doing 2 sets of 4 to 6 reps. Limit yourself to two exercises per muscle group. Beginning with your second month, add a third exercise for each muscle group, and a third set. This may seem like a lot of work, but it should only take you about one hour to complete.

Intermediate Weight-Training Program

Warm-Up

- Five minutes of a light aerobic activity
- One stretching exercise for each muscle group (see Chapter Four)

Shoulders

- Upright Row (Barbell)
- Shoulder Press Machine (Front)
- Shoulder Press Machine (Behind the Neck)
- Side Laterals Machine

Back

- Rowing (Dumbbells)
- Pull Downs

Chest

- Bench Press Machine
- Pullover (Barbell)
- Incline Bench Press Machine
- Peck Deck Machine

Triceps

- Triceps Push Down
- French Curl
- Cable Kick Back
- Cable Triceps Push Down

Biceps

- Preacher Curl
- Standing Cable Curl
- Concentrated Cable Curl

Legs

- Leg Extension
- Leg Curl
- One-Legged Calf Raise
- Leg Press
- Hack Squat

Abdominals

- See Chapter Eight — Intermediate Program

Aerobics

- 20 to 45 minutes at 65 percent to 85 percent of your maximum heart rate, 3 to 5 days per week

Cool-Down

- Five minutes of a light aerobic activity

Routine

Perform 3 sets of 10 to 12 reps, 3 times per week (with a day of rest between sessions). After your first month, add a fourth leg exercise (those with an asterisk). If you want to build muscle, increase the weight and decrease your reps to 8 to 10. If you want to reduce your size, decrease the weight and increase your reps to 12to 15.

Advanced Weight-Training Program

DAY ONE (UPPER BODY)

Warm-Up

- Five minutes of a light aerobic activity
- One stretching exercise for each muscle group (see Chapter Three)

Shoulders

- Shoulder Press Machine (Front)
- Shoulder Press Machine (Behind the Neck)
- Side Laterals Machine
- Pulley Side Laterals

Back

- Narrow (or Wide) Grip Chin-Up
- Seated Rowing Machine
- Pull Downs (Front and Back)

Chest

- Bench Press Machine
- Incline Bench Press Machine
- Flyes (Dumbbells)
- Peck Deck Machine
- Chest Victory Cable Machine

Triceps

- Tricep Extension (Dumbbells)
- Tricep Push Down
- Cable Kick Back
- Cable Triceps Push Down

Biceps

- Concentrates Dumbbell Curl
- Preacher Curl
- Standing Cable Curl

Aerobics

- 30 to 50 minutes at 65 percent to 85 percent of your maximum heart rate, 3 to 5 days per week

Cool-Down

- Five minutes of a light aerobic activity

DAY TWO (LEGS AND ABDOMINALS)

Warm-Up

- Five minutes of a light aerobic activity
- One stretching exercise for each muscle group (see Chapter Four)

Legs

- Leg Extension
- Leg Curl
- Leg Press
- Hack Squat
- Two-Legged Calf Raise
- Seated Calf Raise

Abdominals

- See Chapter Nine — Advanced Program

Aerobics

- 30 to 50 minutes at 65 percent to 85 percent of your maximum heart rate, 3 to 5 days per week

Cool-Down

- Five minutes of a light aerobic activity

Routine

If you want to get yourself into great shape, use what I call the Two-On, One-Off Routine (or Split-day Workout). On the first day you do all upper-body exercises, performing 3 sets of 8 to 10 repetitions. On the second day you do all leg and abdominal exercises, performing 3 sets of 10 to 12 repetitions. Rest on the third day. On your last set, work the muscle to the point of complete exhaustion by doing as many reps as you can. Don't rest more than 30 seconds between exercises.

SHOULDERS

Upright Row (Barbell)

While standing, grasp a barbell with your hands spaced next to each other, knuckles facing away from your body. Pull the bar up to your chin and allow your elbows to extend outward to the sides of your body to help build your shoulders. Lower to thigh level. This is a great exercise for men, but especially for women, who typically have fat pockets in their deltoids and trapezius muscles.

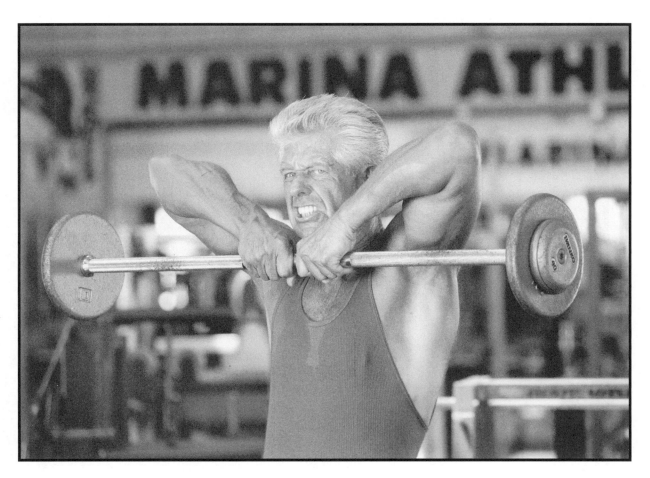

Upright Row (Barbell)

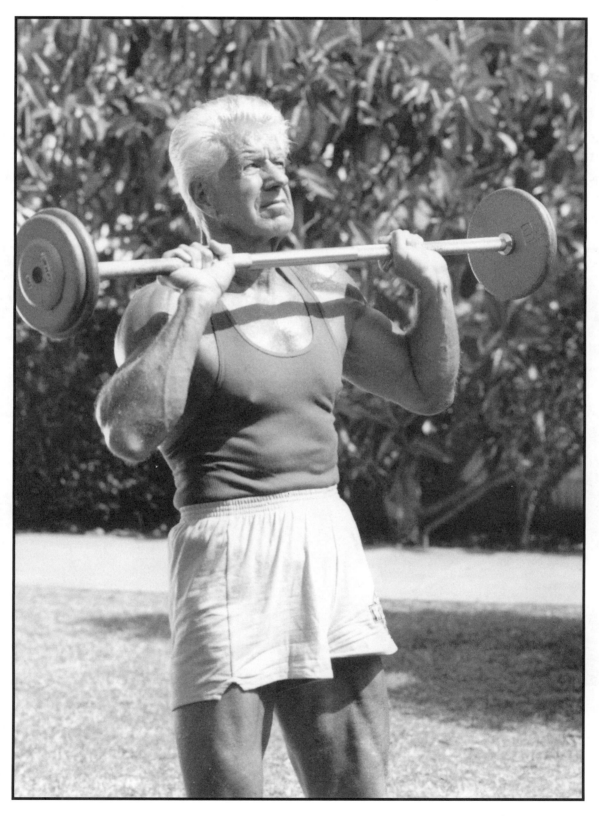

Standing Shoulder Press (Barbell)

Standing Shoulder Press (Barbell)

Grasp the barbell with your hands about shoulder-width apart and your knuckles facing away from your body. Your feet should be comfortably apart. Raise the bar to your chest, flipping your knuckles so that they almost touch your shoulders. Your palms should be facing out from your body, and your eyes looking straight ahead. Press the bar over your head, and return it to chest level. Press up again and return. This exercise puts a lot of pressure and strain on your lower back, so if you have aback problem, wear a weight-training belt. The motion should be fluid, not jerky. Don't arch your back. If you have to cheat, the weight is too heavy.

Seated Shoulder Press (Dumbbells)

Sit at the end of your bench with a dumbbell in each hand. Raise the dumbbells to your chest so that your palms are facing away from your body. Press the dumbbells over your head, and return them to chest level. Press up again and return. Concentrate on working the front deltoid muscles.

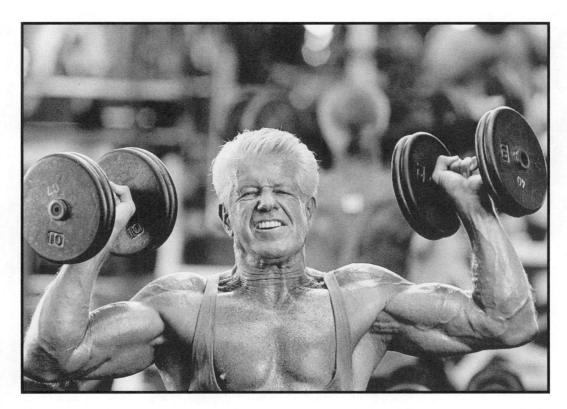

Seated Shoulder Press (Dumbbells)

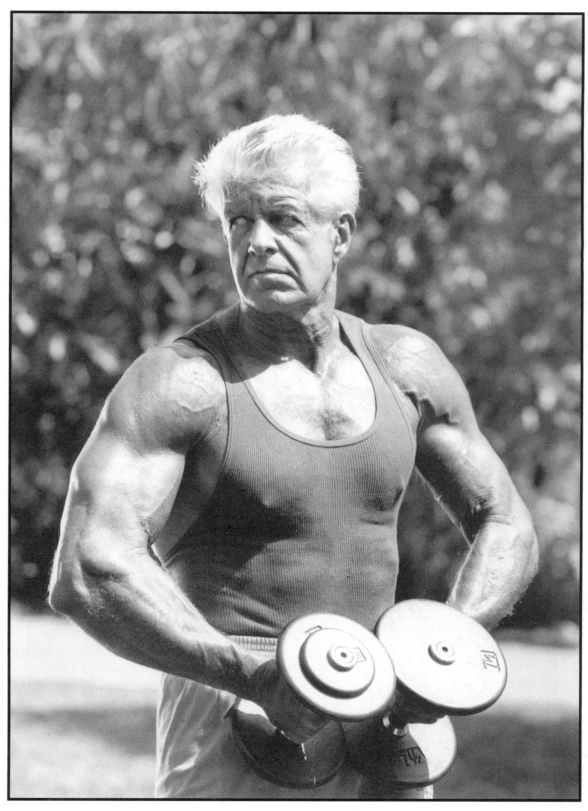

Side Laterals (Dumbbells)

Side Laterals (Dumbbells)

Hold a set of light dumbbells at your side, palms toward your thighs, knuckles facing away from your body. Your elbows should be slightly bent. Raise the dumbbells simultaneously to a vertical position away from your body, and return. Imagine holding two milk cartons and raising them to your side to pour yourself two glasses of milk. This exercise builds the side deltoid muscles that wrap around your shoulders and arms.

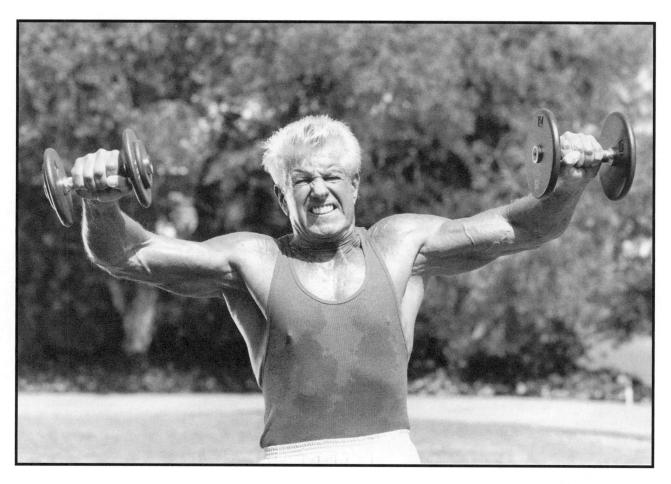

Side Laterals (Dumbbells)

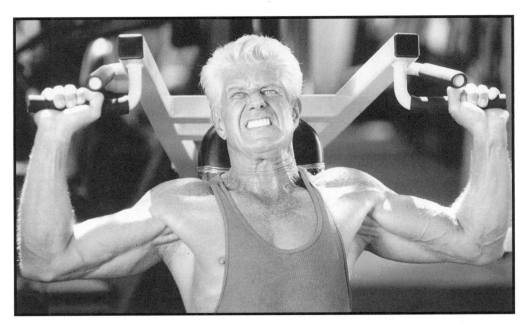

Shoulder Press Machine (Front)

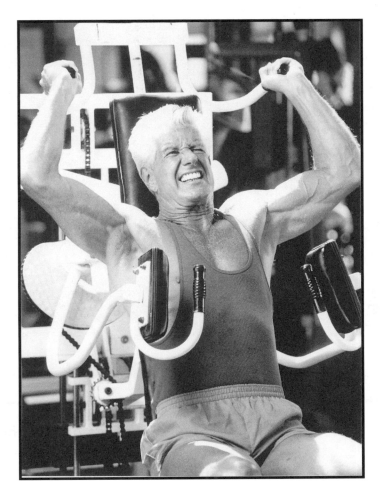

*Shoulder Press Machine
(Behind the Neck)*

Shoulder Press Machine (Front)

Adjust the seat of the machine to fit your body frame. Your shoulders should be aligned with the arms. Grasp the handles of the machine near your shoulders, palms facing away from your body. Keep your back straight. Slowly straighten your arms and push the handles upward toward the ceiling. Once you reach the peak position,slowly lower the handles back to the starting position near your shoulders. This movement works the front deltoids.

Shoulder Press Machine (Behind the Neck)

Adjust the seat to your body frame so that your shoulders are level with the rotation points. Grasp the handles at shoulder level and press the bar straight over your head. Slowly lower the unit behind your neck and press up again to work the back deltoids. Don't use a weight that's too heavy because this exercise puts a lot of pressure on your lower back.

Side Laterals Machine

Adjust the seat so that when you sit down your shoulders are flush with the rotation points of the machine. Place the backs of your wrists against the movement pads of the machine and lightly grasp the handles. Raise the handles sideways away from your body using your deltoids. Keep your elbows above the level of your hands throughout the movement. When you've reached the peak level, slowly lower your hands back to the starting position.

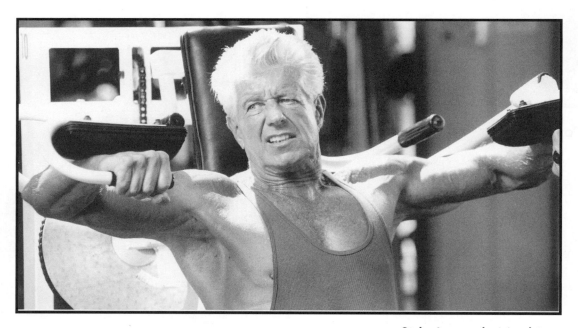

Side Laterals Machine

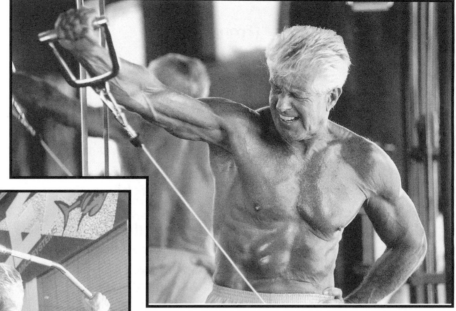

Pulley Side Laterals

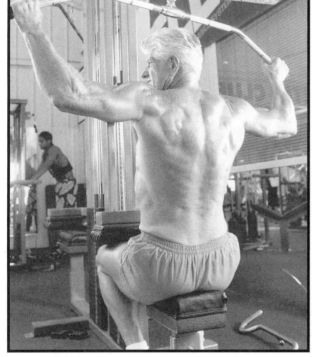

Pull Downs

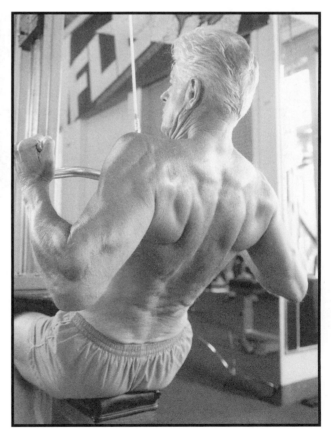

Pull Downs

Pulley Side Laterals

Attach a loop handle to a floor pulley and grab the handle in your right hand, palm up, so that the cable runs diagonally across your body. Allow the weight of the cable machine to pull your right hand across your midsection. Slowly raise your hand across your body to the right, lifting upward until it reaches shoulder level. Hold for a split second and feel the muscle strain. Lower your hand slowly back to the starting point. Be sure not to straighten your arm fully when you reach the finish position, because you want to keep your triceps out of the movement. This exercise also works the deltoids.

BACK

Pull Downs

Take hold of the lat machine bar with your palms facing away from your body and your hands about shoulder-width apart on each side. Sit on the bench and wedge your knees under the restraining bar. Allow the weight of the overhead bar to fully straighten your arms above your head. Slowly bend your arms to pull the bar down behind your neck working the latissimus dorsi muscles. Make sure your elbows travel down and back. Contract the back muscles and arch your back. Slowly return to starting position.

You can perform a number of variations on this exercise. For example, you can change the width of your grip, do the movement with your palms facing toward your body instead of away from your body, or pull the lat bar to your upper chest instead of behind your neck. Experiment on your own.

Rowing (Dumbbells)

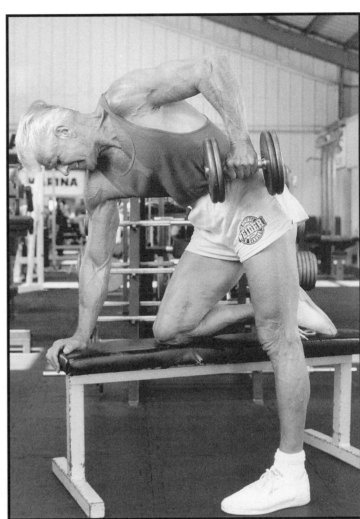

Seated Rowing Machine

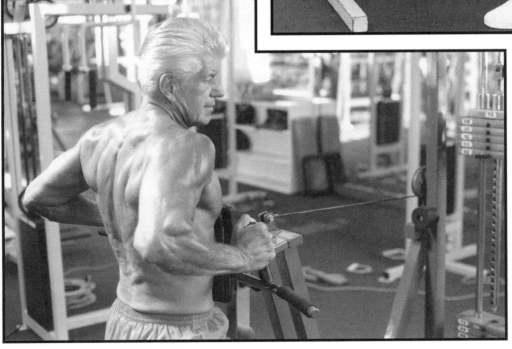

Rowing (Dumbbells)

Place your right knee on the bench, with your left foot on the floor for balance. Using a lightweight dumbbell in your left hand, drop the arm down full length to the floor and pull back up to chest level. This is a great exercise if you want that V-shape. It also helps reduce the fat pockets around your upper back

Seated Rowing Machine

Attach a double-hand grip to the cable and grasp with both hands, palms facing each other. Elevate the seat to a point where you can pull the grip to your lower abdominal muscles. Sit on the padded board of the machine and place your feet against the restraining bar. Bend your legs slightly and allow the weight of the machine to pull you forward, stretching your lats and lower back muscles. Pull the handle toward your torso and up to your abdomen. Keep your elbows tucked against your sides, and your chest out. At the peak of the movement, arch your back slightly, holding the position for a split second, then slowly return to starting position.

Narrow-Grip Chin-Up

Grab a chin-up bar, placing your hands slightly less than shoulder-width apart. Pull yourself up and over the bar, hold for a second, then let yourself down to full length, working the back and arms. To do this exercise at home, you may have to buy a chin-up bar for your doorway. Be sure it is well mounted and tightly secured.

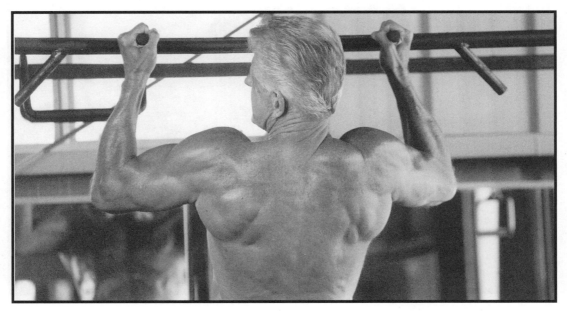

Narrow-Grip Chin-up

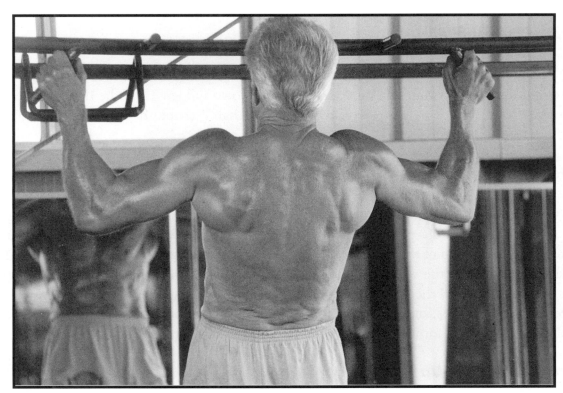

Wide-Grip Chin-Up

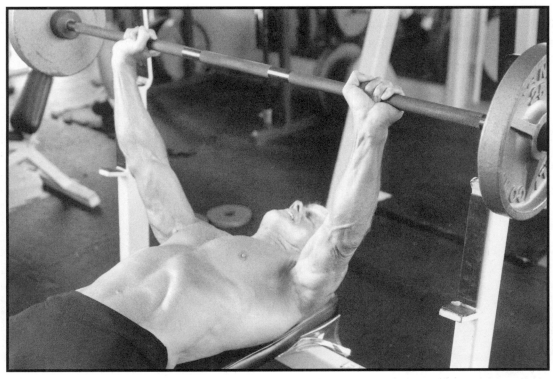

Bench Press (Barbell)

Wide-Grip Chin-Up

Grab a chin-up bar as wide as the bar will permit with your palms facing away from you. Pull yourself up over the bar, hold for a second, then slowly let yourself down to full length. Don't attempt this exercise unless you're confident in your strength and ability.

CHEST

Bench Press (Barbell)

Lie on your back on an exercise bench with your feet flat on the floor. Hold the barbell with your hands slightly more than shoulder-width apart, palms facing away from you. Slowly lower the bar to your chest, hold for a split second, then push it straight up until your arms are fully extended and your elbows almost locked. Let it return to your chest and push it up again. Keep your eyes to the ceiling, and don't arch your back or bounce the weight on your chest. Be sure to breathe correctly by exhaling with the actual bench press, and inhaling on return. If you're using heavy weights, be sure you've got a spotter — someone to stand behind you to catch the weight in case you get into trouble.

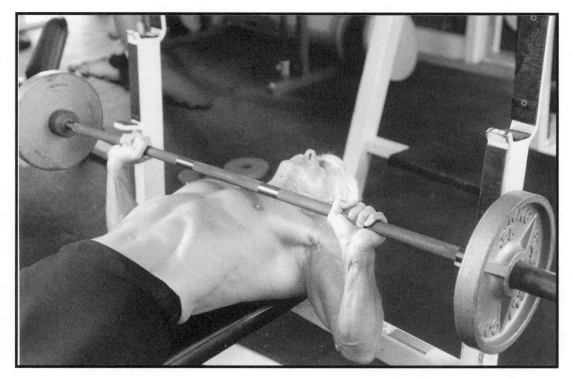

Bench Press (Barbell)

Flyes (Dumbbells)

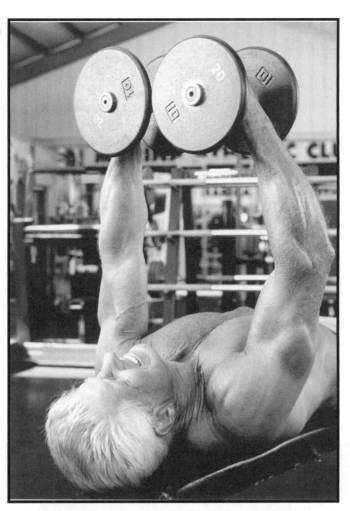

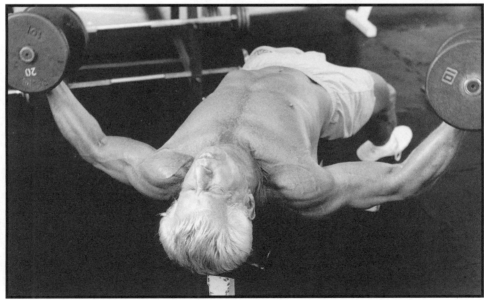

Flyes (Dumbbells)

Bench Press Machine

The Bench Press Machine is a great starting point for those of you who have never used free weights. It works on the same principle as the bench press, except it has a fixed weight stack and pressing bar, which lower your risks and make it easier to use. Lie on your back on the bench with your feet flat on the floor. Grab the pressing bar by the handles, palms facing away from you. Lower the bar to your chest, hold for a split second, then push it straight up until your arms are fully extended and your elbows almost locked. And don't bounce the weight off your chest. Use the same breathing technique that you use with the regular bench press.

Flyes (Dumbbells)

Lying on your back, take a dumbbell in each hand, palms facing each other. Bend your elbows comfortably at bench level. Slowly raise the dumbbells above your chest, squeezing the pectoral muscles, then lower the dumbbells again to bench level.

Incline Chest Press (Dumbbells)

Lie on your back on a slant board or readjust your bench to a 45 degree angle. Hold the dumbbells with your hands about shoulder-width apart, palms out, as if you were going to do a bench press. Slowly lower the dumbbells to your chest, and push them straight up and out from your chest until your arms are fully extended and your elbows almost locked. Pinch together your pectoral muscles, then return the dumbbells to your chest and push them up again. This exercise fills out the upper pectoral muscles.

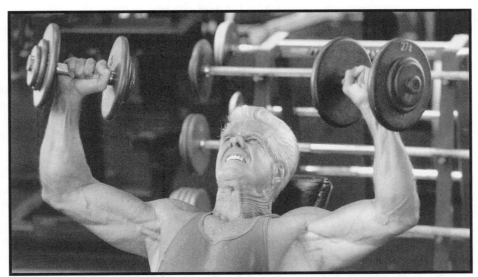

Incline Chest Press (Dumbbells)

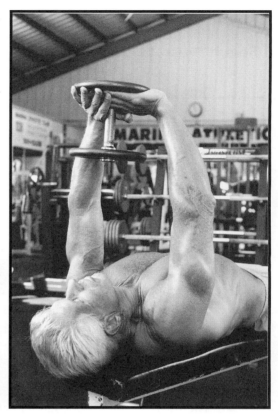

Pullover

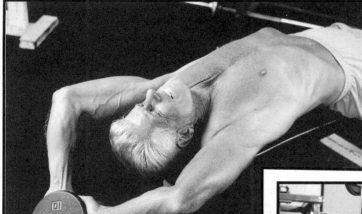

Pullover

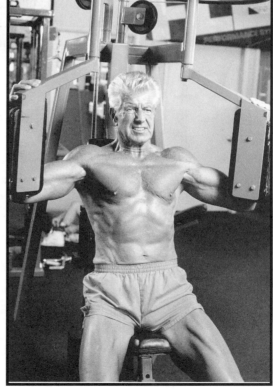

Peck Deck Machine

Pullovers

Be sure to use lighter weights on this exercise, because heavy weights will strain the shoulder joints. Lie on your back on a bench and grasp a dumbbell around the plate. Raise the dumbbell straight up in a semicircular motion and lower it at arms length behind you, expanding the rib cage and lung cavity, and taking in as much oxygen as you can. Bring it back to a vertical-arms position. Besides helping you take in more oxygen, this exercise improves your posture.

Incline Bench Press Machine

Sit down and adjust the seat. Grasp the handles of the machine with your hands about shoulder-width apart, palms out, and press up and out toward the sky, as if you were doing a bench press. Contract the upper pectoral muscles, and return the bar to shoulder level. You can do the same exercise with dumbbells.

Peck Deck Machine

Adjust the seat of the machine. Sit in the seat and force your elbows behind the two rotating pads. Your forearms should be held perpendicular to the floor and your fingers should be resting over the top edges of the pads. Allow your elbows to move as far to the rear as comfortably possible. Working the pectoral muscles, move the pads forward and inward until they kiss each other in front of your chest. Hold for peak contraction and return the pads to the starting position.

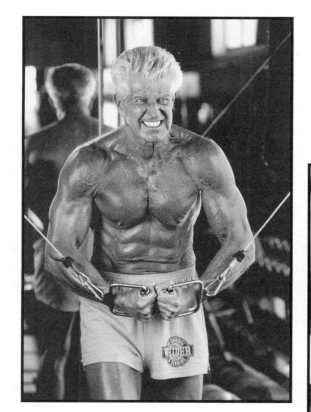

Chest Victory Cable Machine

Triceps Extension (Dumbbells)

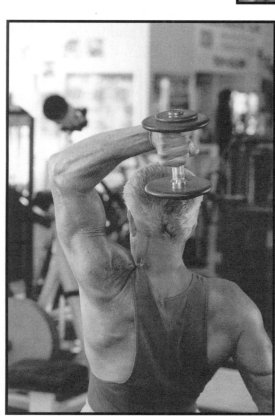

Triceps Extension (Dumbbells)

Chest Victory Cable Machine

Attach two loop handles to the overhead pulleys. Stand with feet about shoulder-width apart between the pulleys and grasp each handle, palms facing toward the floor. Allow the weight of the machine to pull your arms apart. Readjust your feet for proper balance by placing one foot slightly ahead of the other, and arch your back. Slowly pull your hands downward and inward in semicircular arcs until they kiss each other in front of your midsection. Concentrate on really flexing your chest with the movement. Hold for peak contraction, tensing your pectoral muscles and deltoids, then return to starting position. Cable crossovers are a great way to shape and define the lower pectoral muscles.

TRICEPS

Triceps Extension (Dumbbells)

Hold one dumbbell in your left hand and raise your arm over your head. Keeping your arm stationary, bend your elbow and slowly lower the dumbbell behind your neck and raise it back up to the vertical position to work the triceps. Your form is extremely important. Few people do this exercise correctly. Keep a slow, steady pace, and keep your elbow next to your head. If you have to hold your elbow with your other hand to keep it stationary, do so.

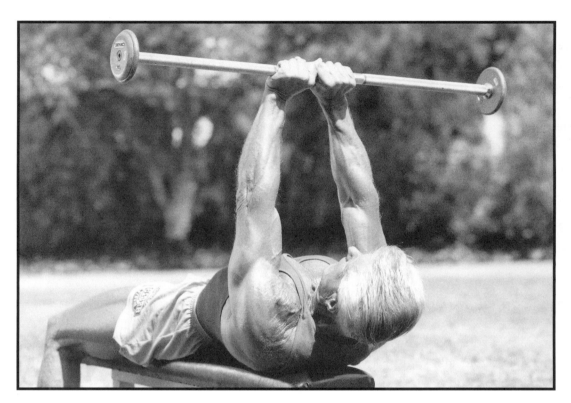

French Curl

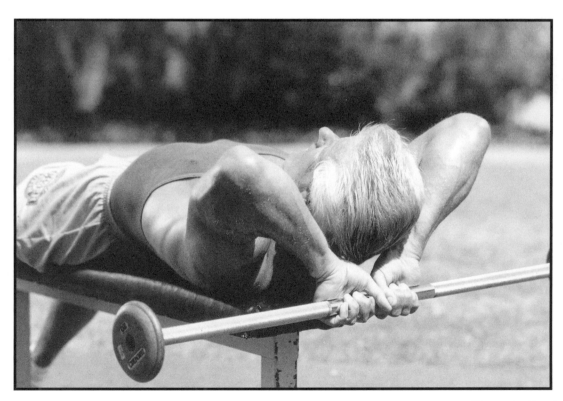

French Curl

Triceps Extension (Barbell)

Hold the barbell with your hands spaced only a few inches apart. Raise the barbell over your head and, keeping your arm stationary, bend your elbows and slowly lower the barbell behind your neck and back up to the starting position.

French Curl

Lie on your back on a bench. Grasp a barbell in the middle, and raise it above your chest. Keeping your arms stationary, lower the barbell behind your head and below the rim of the bench, then back up to the original position. Feel the burning sensation in your triceps. Try to keep your elbows tucked in to reduce the strain on your joints.

Kick Back (Dumbbells)

Place your left knee on the bench, keeping your right foot on the floor for balance. Using a lightweight dumbbell in your right hand, extend your right arm up and behind your back, and lower it back down to the starting position. Keep your arm stiff. If you can't do this without cheating, take off some weight. You need to concentrate on isolating the tricep. I can't do more than 20 pounds on this particular exercise. You really have to exercise the tricep hard to get results.

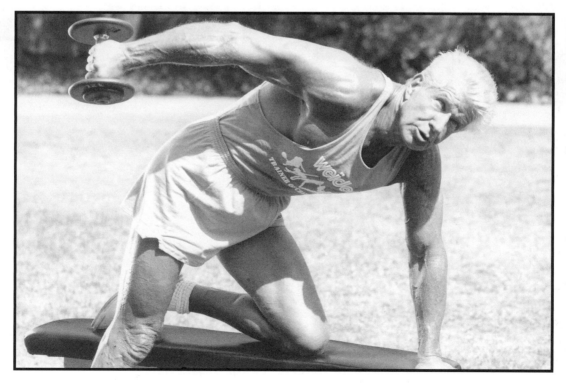

Kick Back (Dumbbells)

Triceps Push Down

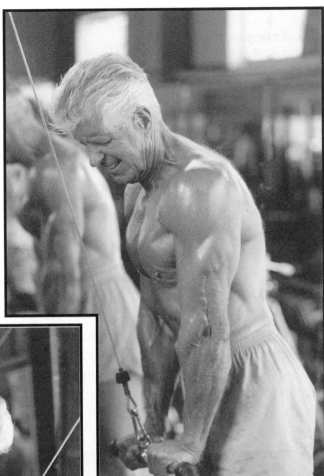

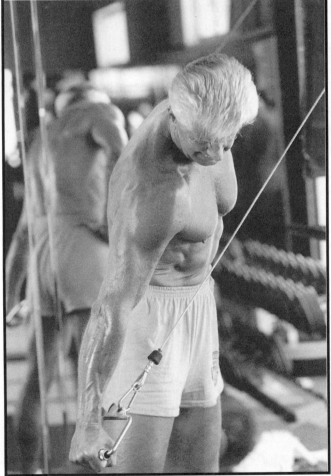

Cable Triceps Push Down

Triceps Push Down

Attach a handlebar to the lat machine. Stand with your feet shoulder-width apart, facing the machine, and grasp the handle with both hands, no more than 3 inches apart, palms away from your body. Your arms should be bent, elbows tucked next to your body. Slowly straighten your arms by pushing the handle down in a semicircular motion. Touch the handle to your upper thighs, and lean into the movement to feel the extension; hold for peak contraction. Concentrate on working the triceps. Return the handle to the starting position.

Cable Kick Back

Attach a loop handle to the lower pulley and grasp the handle with your right hand. Face the machine and stand back roughly 2 feet. Bend at the waist so that your torso is at a 45 degree angle to the floor. Extend your right forearm up and behind your back. Use only your triceps and slowly return the handle to the starting position. Remember, form is important in this exercise.

Cable Triceps Push Down

Attach a loop handle to an overhead pulley and grab it with one hand. With your feet shoulder-width apart and facing the pulley machine, bend your elbow so that the back of your hand is near your shoulders, palms facing away from your body. Slowly straighten your arm, pushing downward and out. Keep your elbow tucked neatly against your torso. Return the handle to the starting position, and repeat to the other side. This exercise works the outer head of the triceps muscles.

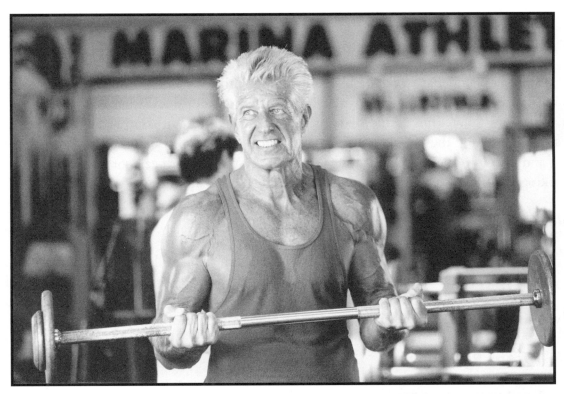

Barbell Curl

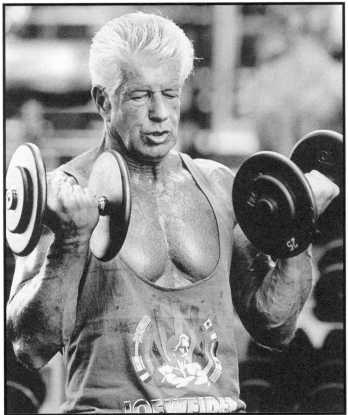

Seated Dumbbell Curl

BICEPS

Barbell Curl

Hold the barbell with your hands spaced about 18 inches apart, palms facing up. The bar should be resting on your upper thighs. Using the muscles in your wrists and arms, curl the bar up to the chest, just below your chin. Do not bend the wrist. Return to starting position. Keep your back straight and your elbows tucked close to your sides. Concentrate on isolating the biceps. If you can't do this without cheating — pushing your elbows out from your sides or arching your buttocks — take off some weight.

Seated Dumbbell Curl

Hold one dumbbell in each hand, palms facing up. The dumbbells should be resting on your upper thighs. Curl the dumbbells up to the chest, just below your chin, again using your wrists and arms, and try to touch the dumbbells to your shoulders. Return to starting position.

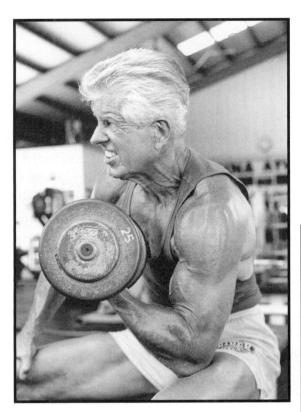

Concentrated Dumbbell Curl

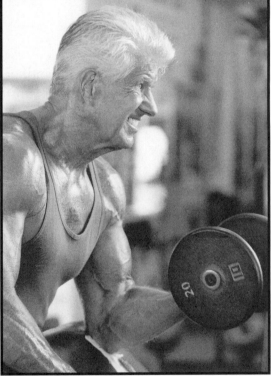

Preacher Curl

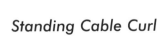

Standing Cable Curl

Concentrated Dumbbell Curl

Sit down and, leaning forward, place your left elbow on your left thigh. The dumbbell should be in your left hand, and your elbow should be resting on your leg with your arm extended toward the center of your body. Curl the dumbbell up until your forearm almost touches your biceps to "peak out" your biceps. Slowly lower the dumbbell to the starting position. Don't jerk or swing the dumbbell. Use proper form. Repeat the same exercise with your right side.

Preacher Curl

Grab a dumbbell and lean over the preacher bench (the preacher bench is basically an incline bench with padding — if you don't have a preacher bench, you can always use the incline bench) so that the padded shelf is wedged under your arms. Straighten your arm down the surface of the shelf (but not to full extension) and slowly curl your arm, bringing the dumbbell up to your chin. Return to starting position. All curls work the biceps muscles. The Preacher Curl, in particular, works the lower part of the biceps where it connects with the forearm near the elbow.

Standing Cable Curl

Attach a loop handle to a floor pulley and grasp it with your right hand. Stand up straight and allow your right arm to extend down the side of your body. With your palm facing away from your body, slowly curl your right hand up and try to touch the loop handle to your right shoulder. Keep your elbow tucked tightly against your body and work the full range of motion of your biceps. Hold for a split second, concentrating on a contracting the muscle, and return to the starting position. Repeat with your left arm. Be sure to isolate the muscle. This is a great exercise for further sculpting the natural formation of your biceps.

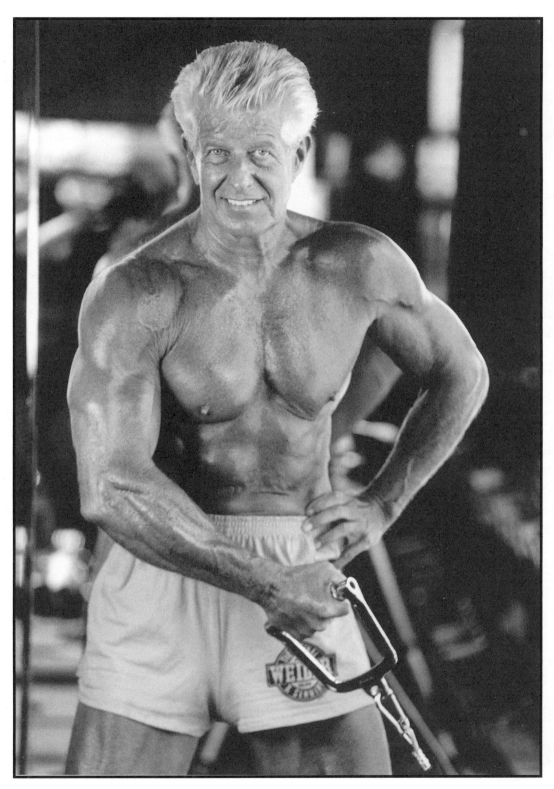

Concentrated Cable Curl

Concentrated Cable Curl

This is the same as the Standing Cable Curl, only this time squat slightly and instead of curling your right hand up to touch your right shoulder, curl it across your body and try to touch the loop handle to your left shoulder. Concentrate on keeping your elbow next to your body and work the full range of motion of your biceps. Hold at peak contraction, then return to starting position. Repeat with the left arm.

LEGS

Half-Squats

Stand erect and hold a lightweight barbell across your shoulders behind your neck. Squat slowly until your thighs are about parallel and seat level to the floor. Keep your upper body straight as you return to the upright position just short of knee lock (to keep tension on your thighs). It's a good idea to put a bench or chair behind you so that when you reach the half-squat position your buttocks will hit the bench and you can't go down too far.

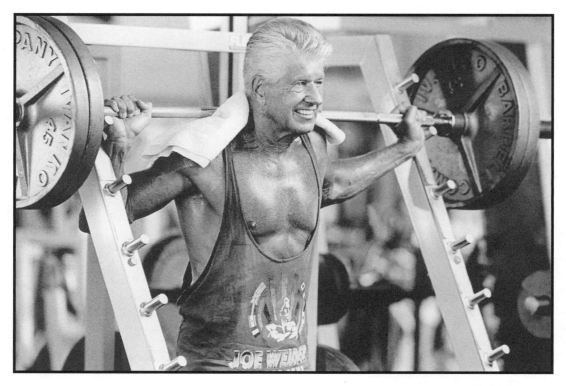

Half-Squats

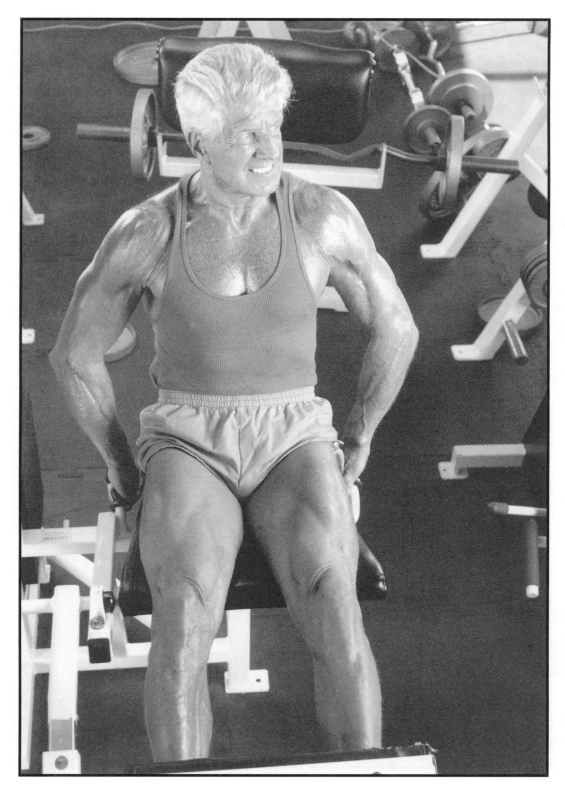

Leg Extension

Leg Extension

Sit on the end of the leg extension machine and hook your ankles under the weights. Hold the edges of the bench with both hands and extend your knees so that they are parallel to the floor. Hold for a split second, then release slowly. Muscle is built on the down stroke, so a smooth slow rhythm is important.

Leg Curl

Lie on your stomach on the leg extension machine and hold on to the bench. Hook your feet beneath the weight bar and, lifting your feet behind you, try to touch your buttocks with your heels. Hold for a split second, then slowly lower your legs back to the original position. Don't bounce.

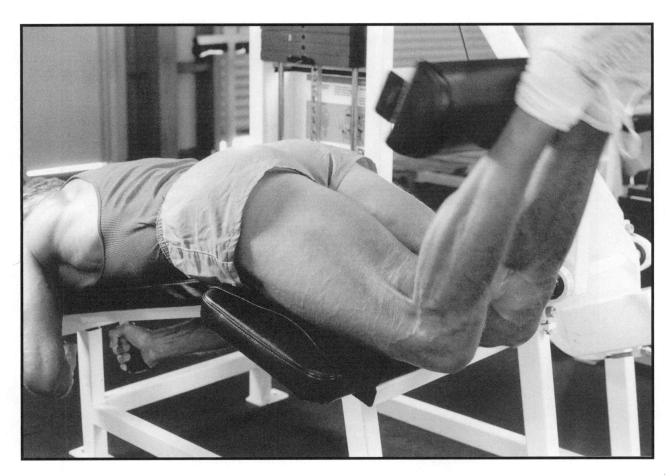

Leg Curl

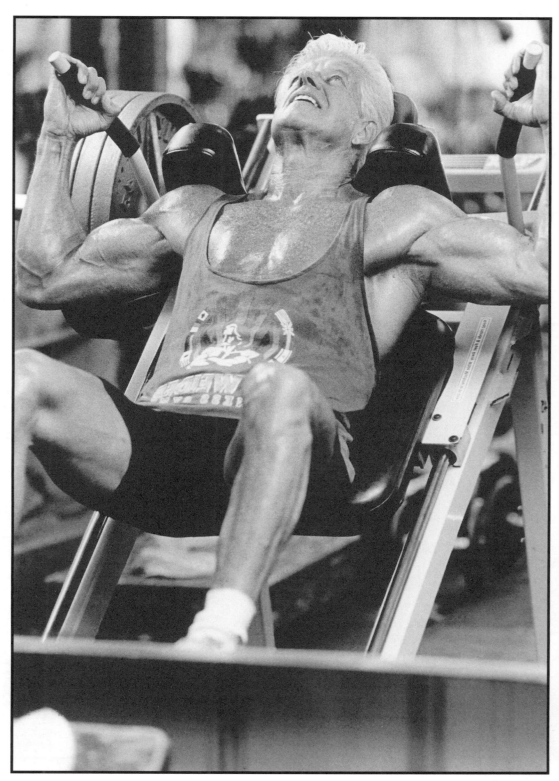

Hack Squat

Hack Squat

Place your body on the hack machine so that the pads fit snugly over your shoulders. From the upright position, fully bend your legs down to the "squatting" position and feel the tension in your thigh muscles and the quadriceps just above your knees. Slowly straighten your legs to within 6 inches of the fully straight position.

Leg Press

Adjust the seat of the leg press machine to fit your body frame. Sit on the seat and place your feet on the pedals. Grasp the handles at the sides of the seat and keep your arms and spinal column straight as you slowly straighten your legs. Once your knees are nearly locked out, slowly bend your legs down, then back up. If you're looking for an even tougher workout, try performing the same exercise by starting in the down position and coming up halfway.

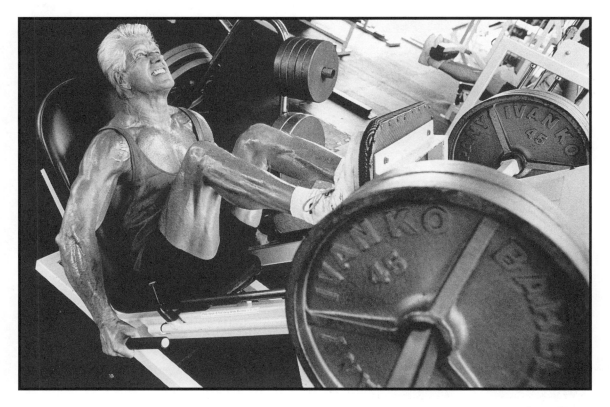

Leg Press

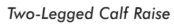

Two-Legged Calf Raise

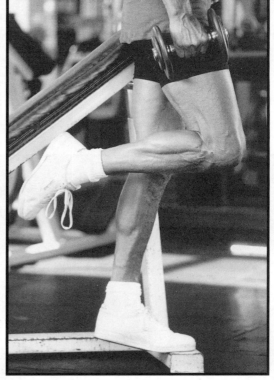

One-Legged Calf Raise

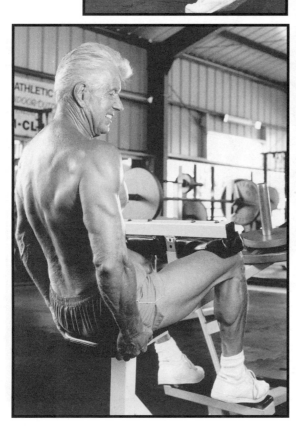

Seated Calf Raise

Two-Legged Calf Raise

Stand straight, with feet shoulder-width apart and the barbell resting comfortably behind your neck and on your shoulders. Keeping your back straight, and without bending your legs, rise up on your toes, and back down. This exercise can also be done without weights if you're not quite ready to intensify your workout.

One-Legged Calf Raise

With a dumbbell in one hand, stand with the ball of your foot on a 2x4 piece of board. If the dumbbell is in your right hand, stand on your right foot, and vice versa. Support yourself with your other hand against a wall or by holding on to a chair or table. Keeping your back straight and without bending your right leg, rise up on your toes as high as you can, hold for a split second, then lower yourself, stretching the calf muscles. Do as many as you can. If you choose, this exercise can also be done without weights.

Seated Calf Raise

Sit on the seat of the machine so that your toes and the balls of your feet are on the toe bar and your knees are tucked snugly underneath the pads. As you did for the standing calf raises, rise up on your toes as high as you can, then lower yourself, stretching the calf muscles. Do as many as you can. You may want to change the position of your feet from toes pointing forward, to toes pointing either inward or outward.

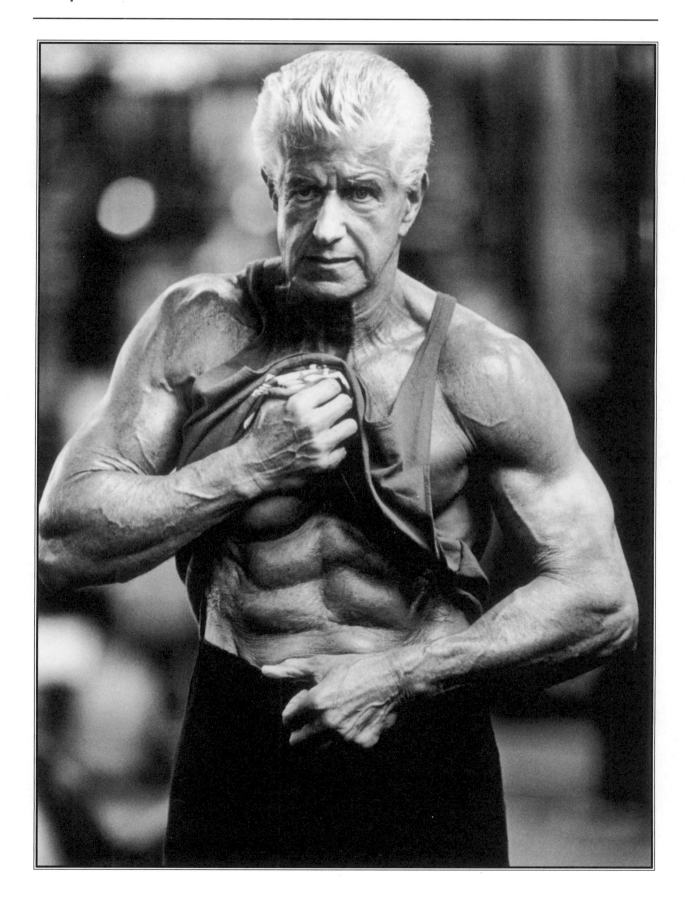

Developing Strong Abdominal Muscles

Your waist line is your life line.

A soft midsection can be one of the first signs that middle age is creeping up on you, and it's typically the hardest area to keep trim. More importantly — excess weight around one's chest and waist have been linked to breast cancer in women and heart disease in men. A study at the University of Minnesota, however, found that women ages 55 to 69 who have an "apple" shape — a bigger waist than hips — have the same high risk of death that men of this shape exhibit. To put it quite simply, your waistline is your lifeline. But you won't be able to tone those abdominals without first understanding a few of the fundamentals.

Developing a firm and tight waistline and a detailed torso depends on a lot more than just sit-ups. Most people have a layer of fat around their stomachs. All the abdominal exercises in the world won't get rid of that layer of fat; the only effective way to lose excess abdominal fat and build rock-hard abs is with a low-fat diet and a regular aerobics program (30 minutes, 3 to 4 days per week). People who perform ab exercises without addressing the problem of excess stomach fat may develop well toned abdominal muscles, but the results won't be visible. Look at sumo wrestlers. They do 5,000 sit-ups a day, but they've got 60 inch waistlines. It's all in the diet.

The abdominals are arranged in crisscrossing layers that are divided into upper and lower segments. The upper segment draws your rib cage toward your pelvis, while the lower segment draws your pelvis toward your rib cage. For training purposes, we will call these the *upper* and *lower abs*. Lower-ab movements rely on both upper and lower segments of the muscles, while upper-ab movements rely solely on the upper segments.

The broad, flat muscles wrapping the sides and front of the abdominal region — one of the major fat pockets for men — are called the external obliques. These muscles help the torso bend forward and to the side. There's also a layer of internal obliques, which run at a 90 degree angle to the external obliques. Their main job is to help facilitate twisting motions and compress the abdomen. They also aid the muscles we use when we exhale or cough. There are also muscles that run horizontally across the abdominal region, wrapping around from back to front like a girdle.

Developing a detailed torso takes quality abs as well as strong internal and external oblique muscles. In upper-ab exercise, the torso moves in relation to a stationary pelvis. In lower-ab exercise, the pelvis moves in relation to a stationary torso. The obliques are worked through a variety of twisting motions. Most people don't know how to properly execute movements that work the abdominal muscles and obliques. In fact, most people are wasting their time doing movements that really don't work.

Before I give you the exercises you need to develop hard abs, you need to know which ones are a waste of time. Do not attempt flat and incline bent-knee sit-ups, for example, or straight-legged sit-ups or flat leg raises. These exercises tend to work primarily your hip flexors (which work to balance your torso), not your abdominals. They also put stress on your lower back placing you at a greater risk of injury. The range of motion for the abdominals is roughly 30 degrees. Any movement beyond that will be a waste of time, because you'll be working other muscles.

The different positions and movements of the following exercises help place emphasis on each muscle group in your stomach. A few are aimed at the lower abs, and a few at the upper abs. Others are aimed at the obliques. Contrary to popular belief, you can't "spot reduce" the fat pockets around your obliques, otherwise known as the "love handles." Some exercises that incorporate twisting or bending with light weights actually make the bulges around your sides worse because you end up with oversized obliques. Be patient and the love handles will slowly reduce in size. Remember, though, that reduction of excess fat in the oblique area calls for aerobic and dietary measures, not further development of the oblique muscles.

Abs are some of hardest muscles to train. The key to a proper ab movement is to experience an intense "burning" sensation in the muscle. If you can push yourself beyond the burn and continue to work the muscle, you can increase the efficiency with which you develop abdominal muscles and train with even greater intensity, achieving superior results in less time. The goal, of course, is always to do an exercise with the proper form. Never arch your lower back and never hold your breath. Proper breathing is essential to an effective abdominal workout. Exhale while the muscles are contracting and under maximum stress.

I'm going to show you a number of advanced exercises, but if I were going to do consistently only one exercise for my abdominal muscles, it would definitely be Swedish Breathing. You can do it while driving, cooking even while lying in bed. Roughly 10 times a day will help you keep that waistline trim. By pushing your pelvic area back, it helps improve your posture — which automatically gives you a slimmer look. At the same time, it also firms and tones the midsection.

With your knees slightly bent and your hands on your thighs, inhale deeply, exhale completely. Exhalation is the secret. After all the air has been expelled from your lungs, draw in your

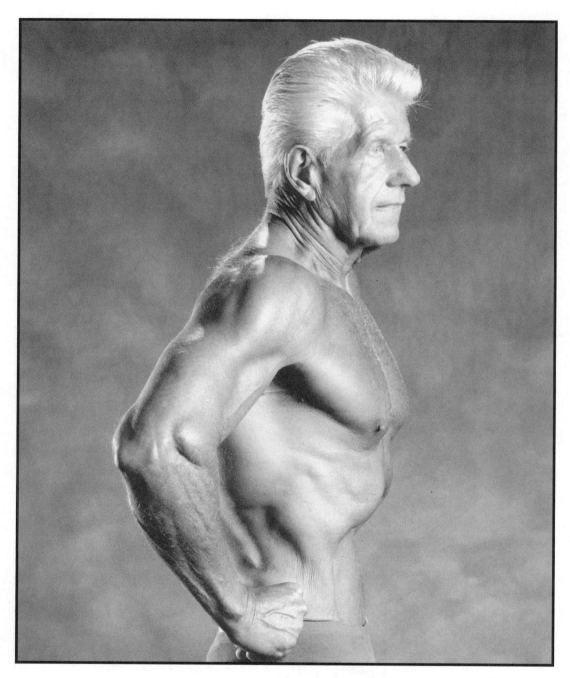

Developing Strong Abdominal Muscles

stomach so that your pubic bone tilts upward into your backbone (this takes a little practice). Hold for a count of 5, then release. After you've mastered the bent-knee version, try performing Swedish Breathing by standing straight up with your hips back and your chest forward. Never do this exercise on a full stomach.

Here are the rest of the exercises you need to develop strong abdominal muscles. You'll find specific training recommendations for each fitness level at the end of the chapter.

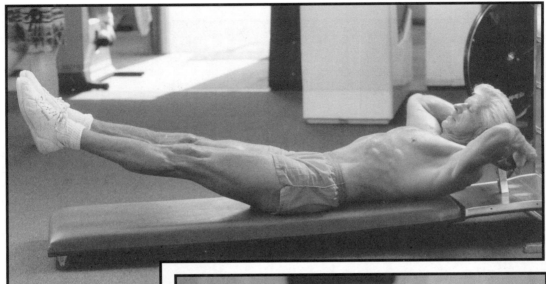

Leg Raise

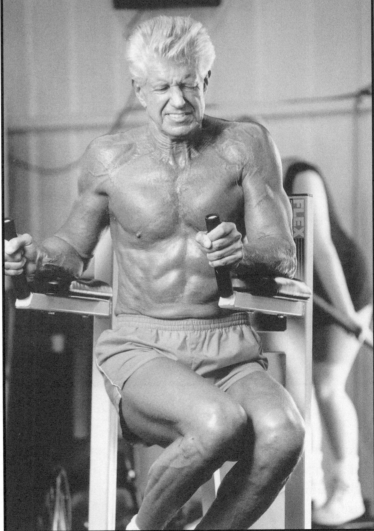

Knee-Up

EXERCISES FOR YOUR LOWER ABS

Leg Raise

Lie down on a carpeted floor. (Nothing good can come from this exercise if your backbone is grinding against a hard surface.) Keep your feet together and legs straight. Raise your feet 18 to 24 inches, never bringing your feet high enough to gain a resting advantage. Lower your feet to within 3 inches of the starting position and hold to strengthen the lower abdominal muscles. Your feet should not come to rest until the end of the exercise. If you experience any discomfort in your back, elevate your head to help keep your lower back from arching, or try doing the exercise one leg at a time.

Knee-Up

Place your hands and elbows on the hand rests of the ab flexor machine. Assume a comfortable position and rock forward using your abdominal muscles to raise your legs to your chest, with your knees bent at a 90 degree angle. Use elbow and/or wrist straps to really work the abdominal muscles instead of the arms or shoulders. Hold at the peak contraction, then slowly lower your body back down to the starting position. Make sure that your abs are doing the work here; a common problem with this exercise is that people use the strength of their arms and shoulders against the knee-up machine to lift their legs rather than forcing the abs to carry the load.

Lying Leg Thrust

Lie on your back on the floor. Elevate your head using your hands for support. Flatten your lower back and raise your hips and legs about 14 to 18 inches off the floor. Keep your knees bent slightly. Rock your pelvis and legs upward until your feet point straight up toward the sky. Imagine a point at which they suddenly hit a wall and the momentum of your legs is deflected upward. Give an upward thrust with your pelvis. Drop straight down, and allow your legs to return to the starting position. Concentrate on fully absorbing the momentum at the bottom of the rep with your abs, not with your back. And try to keep your head and shoulders off the ground. It helps alleviate the pressure on your lower back.

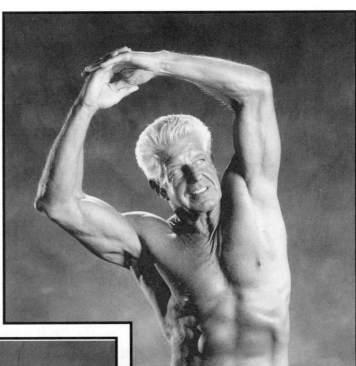

Monkey Side Bend

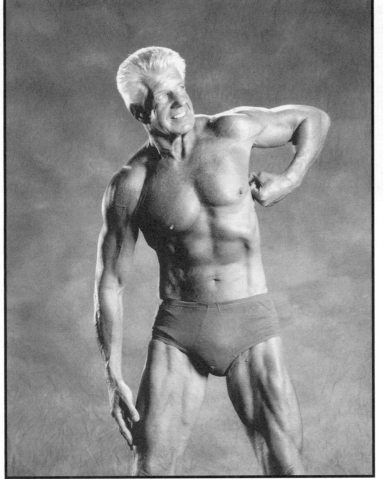

Overhead Side Bend

EXERCISES FOR YOUR UPPER ABS AND OBLIQUES

Overhead Side Bend

This two-way stretching routine burns those stubborn fat pockets (or "love handles") along the sides of your midsection. Clasp your hands and raise them directly over-head. It's important to lean back slightly from the waist. Bend to the right as far as you can without moving your torso forward. Elbows should be bent slightly and pointed toward the floor. Return to erect position and bend to the left for one complete movement. Come to a stop at the erect position each time to be sure you're doing the exercise properly and working those oblique muscles.

Monkey Side Bend

Stand erect with your left palm against your left thigh and your right hand up near your chest. Now bend to the left until your fingertips are just below your left knee. Return to erect position and repeat. Next switch the positions of your hands and bend to the right. Stretch those obliques.

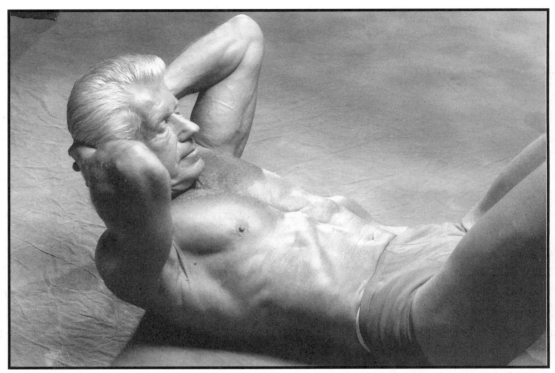

Abdominal Crunch #1

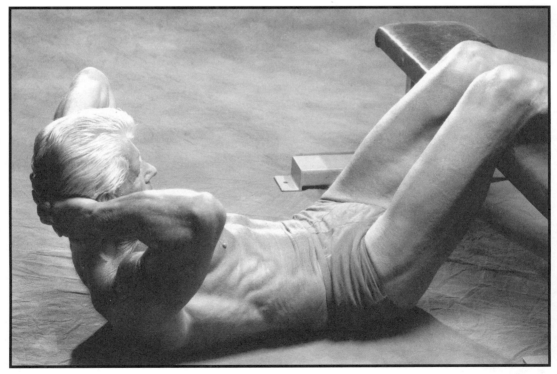

Abdominal Crunch #2

Abdominal Crunch #1

This is the most basic of all stomach exercises, and one of the most misunderstood. Unless the Abdominal Crunch is done properly, it is likely to result in severe muscle strain. Regular sit-ups raise the entire torso so that your knees touch your elbows. But by raising your torso only a short distance from the ground, the rib cage and pelvis draw together, working the abs directly and alleviating lower back problems.

Lie on a soft surface with your knees bent and your feet flat on the floor. Crunch the muscles together by "rolling" your upper body forward. Lifting your shoulder blades off the ground, hold for several seconds, contract the muscles, and move slowly back to starting position. The movement should be short and concise. The harder you contract the muscles the more you're going to get from the exercise.

Abdominal Crunch #2

This exercise is similar to the Abdominal Crunch # 1, with one exception. Lie on your back with knees bent at a 90 degree angle and draped over a chair or bench. But instead of "rolling" your upper body forward, lift your torso and raise your neck and shoulders up, as if to bring your rib cage toward the ceiling. Keep the range of motion short. Another way is to try raising the head, neck and shoulders straight up toward the ceiling, as if a string were attached to your chin.

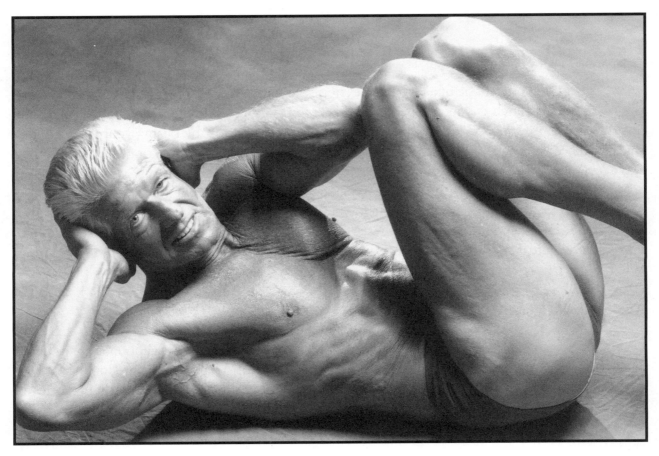

Cross Knee Abdominal Crunch

Cross-Knee Abdominal Crunch

This is a great one for the fat pockets that often appear around the obliques. Lie on your back with knees bent, feet in the air. Place your hands near the side of your neck but not laced together behind your head. With your elbows back, slowly raise your left shoulder and upper back (including your hip), rotate your body about 45 degrees and bring your left shoulder to your right knee.

Concentrate on using your abdominal muscles and not your leg muscles. If you're turning to the right, you should feel the movement somewhere on your left side, running from your ribs down to about your waist. Turn to your left and use your left hand to feel for a contraction in the muscles on your right side. The more twist you can achieve, the more pronounced the contraction. Hold for several seconds at the peak contraction point, then slowly return to the starting position. Repeat on the other side.

Partial Sit-Up

Lie on your back with knees bent and feet in the air so that your hips are directly below your knees Raise your torso just enough to bring your rib cage close to your pelvis, crunching your abs at the top of the movement, then return to the starting position.

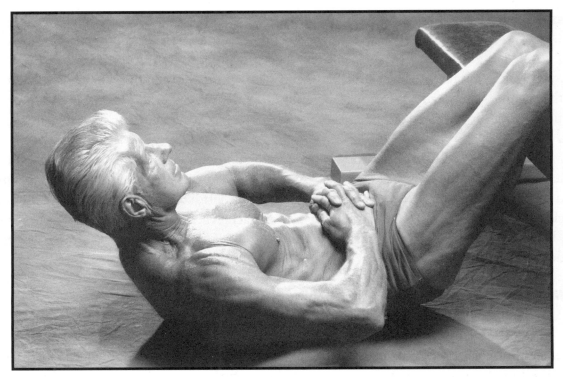

Zane Crunch

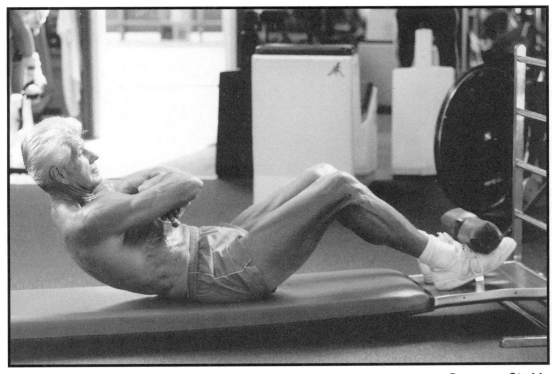

Reverse Sit-Up

Zane Crunch

Frank Zane, three time Mr. Olympia, taught me this one. Lie on your back on the floor with your legs draped across a bench. Fold your hands across your stomach and raise your head, shoulders, and hips as high as you can toward the sky. Contract the stomach muscles at peak level, then slowly lower your body back down to the floor.

Reverse Sit-Up

This is the same as the Zane Crunch, only start at the peak level and slowly lower your body back to the floor about halfway, then back up. Keep your arms crossed in front of you to maintain your balance and rhythm. This is my favorite exercise because it's tough to do, but it really brings out those abs. Keep the tension at all times.

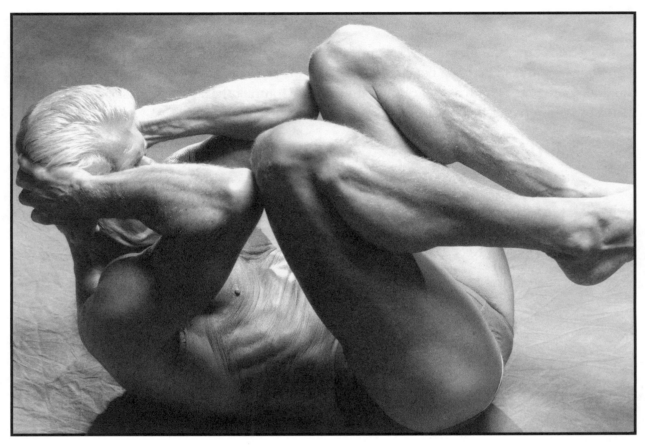

Accordion Sit-Up

Accordion Sit-Up

Lie on your back with knees bent at a 90 degree angle and your feet in the air. Clasp your hands behind your head, and bring your torso to your knees and your knees to your torso at the same time, then release by dropping your torso and knees back to starting position (but not down to the floor).

Beginning	Sets	Reps
Swedish Breathing	1	10
Overhead Side Bend	2	10
Leg Raise	2	10
Abdominal Crunch # 1	2	15

Intermediate	Sets	Reps
Swedish Breathing	1	10
Monkey Side Bend	2	25
Abdominal Crunch #2	2	25
Partial Sit-Up	2	25
Cross-knee Abdominal Crunch	2	25

Advanced	Sets	Reps
Swedish Breathing	1	10
Zane Crunch	2	50
Reverse Sit-Up	2	50
Twisting Accordion Sit-Up	2	50
Knee-Up*	2	15
Lying Leg Thrust	2	50

Routine

Work your way up to the suggested number of exercises. Add repetitions and sets as your muscles get stronger and you become more comfortable with the program. Remember, quality is more important than quantity. You're always better off doing 5 good reps than 50 bad ones. And be sure to take a 15 to 30 second pause between exercises. After a few weeks, you may find that one particular exercise is better than another. Throw away the ones that don't give you that burning sensation anymore, or mix up the routines.

* Interchange with one of the other exercises about once a month.

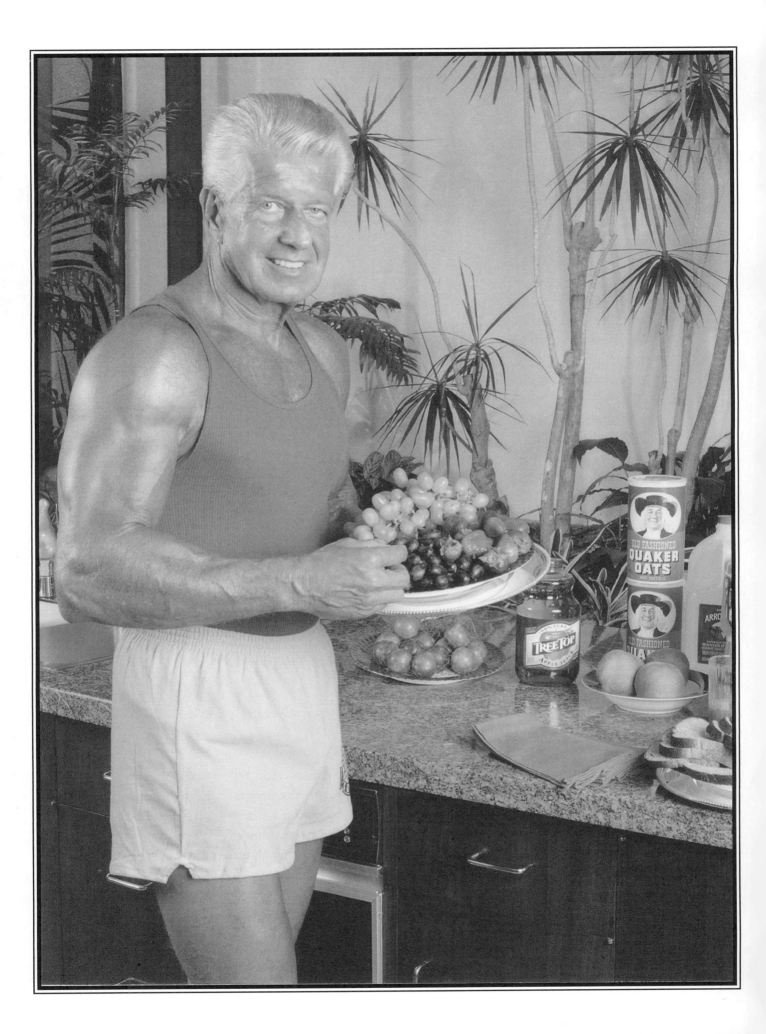

PHASE FOUR:
Nutrition & Longevity

You are what you eat.

In the preceding chapters, I've introduced you to the Isotension, cardiovascular, and weight-training programs that I've developed over years of tinkering with my body and sharing my knowledge with others. But if there's one thing that I've learned, it's that if you really want to lose fat, gain muscle, increase your stamina and strength, and discover the secret to longevity, you must change your eating habits. Unfortunately, few of us have the will power to follow a strictly regimented diet. What we really need is a sensible system of food intake that we can follow forever.

The foundation of your success, however, will depend largely on the relationship between the amount of food you consume and the amount of time you spend exercising. If you want to lose fat and gain muscle, simply abstaining from food is not the answer. Without food, you won't be able to muster the energy to step up your activity. Therefore, you must reorganize your life to include regular exercise and the appropriate diet.

What's an appropriate diet? Try to eat everything as close to nature as possible. That means no preservatives or additives, no salt, butter, or junk food, and it means eating everything in the proper proportions (proteins, carbohydrates, fat, etc.). I'm not saying you've got to drink carrot juice or prepare tofu burgers to stay healthy, but there is one basic truth to losing weight: You gain weight when your body takes in more calories than it uses.

Starting around your twenty-first birthday, things like metabolism (the process by which your body releases energy) and lean muscle mass begin to decrease or diminish, according to the Tufts University research. When people reach 40, they start to suffer from the symptoms of poor nutrition including weight loss dizziness, and loss of appetite. The problem is that the older we get the fewer calories we need, yet we continue to eat as if we're still 20 year-olds. Too many calories and too little exercise, along with a declining metabolic rate, add up to more fat. The Tufts University study concluded that older people's reduced muscle mass is responsible for a 2 percent drop in their basal metabolic rate every 10 years.

Of course, nutrition is not something you should put off until you're 40, especially if you want a trim profile. You need to start paying attention to the details in your life. If you're overweight, for example, it means that you're taking in more food than you're expending in activity, which leaves you with two choices: Exercise more or eat less. The object, of course, is to find a new list of foods that will be satisfying and realistic. And the main idea is not to cut down on the amount of food you eat, but the kind of food you eat.

Every tabloid doctor and diet specialist in the country has a program that claims to magically melt away pounds. You may even know a few television personalities who have gone on record in support of one or two of these programs. I've actually lived my diet for the past 50 years, and I'm the proof that it works. After years of prescribing menus for weight control, I've arrived at a general set of rules on eating. Most of them are as old as common sense — but I've found that plain common sense often vanishes when the mashed potatoes hit the table.

When I talk of diets, by the way, I don't mean a three week, quick-loss program or a pound of diet pills and broccoli. You need to find a program that you can stick with the rest of your life because a lifetime commitment is what it takes A lot of people who start diets end up in the "Yo-Yo Syndrome" — they lose weight one week and gain it all back the next. This is extremely bad for your health since it usually stems from nutritionally unsound advice, and havoc is wreaked on your body as it tries to keep up. Fad diets may work, but at the expense of good health. What you really need is a sensible system of food intake that is not a "diet" at all.

TOTAL DAILY CALORIC INTAKE

Let's start with the fundamentals of a healthy eating plan. Health specialists recommend the following mix of nutrients for middle-aged adults:

Carbohydrates   50-55%

Sources: Fresh fruits, fresh vegetables, whole-grain breads, and starches (potatoes, rice, beans, pasta).

Carbohydrates are the body's main source of energy, and they are crucial nutrients for everyone. They assist in the digestion and assimilation of other foods, and they provide us with immediately available calories for energy. There are two kinds of carbohydrates: simple and complex. Simple carbohydrates are the refined and natural sugars. Most, except those found in fresh fruits and watery vegetables, have no nutritional value and are mostly poison for the body because they have the effect of suddenly raising the insulin level and causing dizziness, nausea, and headaches. So instead of reaching for a candy bar when you're tired, grab a piece of fruit. I eat a piece of fruit every 2 1/2 hours to help keep my energy level at full throttle.

Complex carbohydrates are the grains, cereals, and starches. They're digested slowly and release glucose into the bloodstream gradually, which makes them an ideal source of energy for long workouts. They also contain beneficial vitamins and minerals. Simple carbs, on the other hand, are almost immediately digested into the bloodstream. To lose weight, cut down on complex carbs; bread, potatoes, rice and pasta and cut down on sugary fruit.

Fats   15-20%

Sources: Animal meat, dairy products, hydrogenated and tropical vegetable oils.

Fats are the most concentrated source of energy in the diet. But they also furnish more than twice the number of calories per gram furnished by carbohydrates and proteins. You can't eliminate from your diet all fats for one important reason: Fats help your body absorb several essential vitamins that help your body repair itself from a workout.

Older women, especially, need to watch their fat intake. Eating less saturated fat may reduce your chances of getting breast cancer, according to one study at the Fred Hutchinson Cancer Research Center in Seattle. Scientists there put 73 healthy post-menopausal women on low-fat diets for 12 to 22 weeks. The diets — which cut daily fat intake from an average 68.5 grams to 29.5 grams — also resulted in an average weight loss of 7 1/2 pounds and reduced the women's blood cholesterol by an average of 12 milligrams. Polyunsaturated fats are an important part of your diet. Substitute flax seed oil or olive oil for butter; try adding pumpkin seeds, avocado, pecans, sunflower seeds or almonds to give you the essential fatty acids and Omega 3 & 6 oils your body needs.

Protein   30-35%

Sources: Fish, poultry, lean red meats, low-fat dairy products, eggs, dried beans, protein powder and amino acids. Fish, especially salmon, is my favorite because it gives me protein, my daily dose of Omega 3 and essential fatty acids.

Protein builds everything from muscles and bones to hair and toenails. It is one of the most important elements for the maintenance of good health and vitality. I happen to firmly believe that if you don't get enough protein your body turns to mush. A lot of doctors and nutritionists, however, will tell you not to eat a lot of protein, particularly as you get older. They say it can place too much stress on the kidneys which tend to decline with age. This could be true if you don't exercise and drink enough water.

But, according to a study several years ago by the American College of Sports Medicine, people who exercise several times a week may not be getting enough protein. Research at the Applied Physiology Research Laboratory at Kent State University suggested that protein requirements change dramatically if you exercise. Just 30 minutes of aerobic exercise 3 times a week raises the body's protein need by as much as 25 percent.

So how much protein do you need?

These days, roughly 30 to 35 percent of my daily caloric intake is protein. Another way to look at it is to divide your body weight by two. If you weigh 180 pounds, you should be eating a minimum of 90 grams of protein — if you want to maintain the gains you've made in lean body mass. If you want that rock-hard look, add another 50 percent to your diet; in the case of the 180 pound person, that would be 135 grams of protein. Finally, if you want to build more muscle, eat 1 gram of protein for every pound of body weight. (Be sure to drink plenty of water; it helps wash out the metabolic waste that protein conversion naturally produces.) The thing to focus on is the quality of protein — eat lean sources like lean meat, fish, and low-fat dairy products. I typically choose a 6 ounce can of tuna or a broiled chicken breast (with the skin removed, of course). Each has roughly 40 grams of protein. It's impossible to have a lean, muscular body without the proper amount of protein. But don't eat it all at one meal. Spread it over 3 to 5 times throughout the day. Protein has an almost mystic quality to it; it burns fat, repairs old cells, builds new ones. Without a good supply of protein, your body will turn to mush.

As an added way to increase your protein intake try one of my recipes for protein drinks that are tasty and easily prepared. All you have to do is mix the following ingredients in a blender and serve in a chilled glass.

VITAMIN C COOLER
6 ounces grapefruit or orange juice
1 tablespoon honey
1 teaspoon wheat germ
1 tablespoon protein powder
5 drops lemon juice
1/2 cup crushed ice

STRAWBERRY DELIGHT
10 strawberries (or sliced fresh peach or pineapple)
1 tablespoon protein powder
1 teaspoon wheat germ
6 ounces low-fat milk
2 raw egg whites
1/2 cup crushed ice

THE ENERGIZER
8 ounces nonfat milk
2 tablespoons honey
1 small banana
1 teaspoon brewer's yeast
1 tablespoon protein powder
1 tablespoon wheat germ
1 cup crushed ice

A SENSIBLE PLAN FOR BETTER HEALTH

As soon as you wake up. Warm glass of water with a twist of lemon, and a piece of fresh fruit, either grapefruit or melon. This gives you immediate energy.

Morning. Oatmeal or bran (natural) cereal and nonfat milk. Slice of whole wheat toast (no butter, of course), and coffee or tea. Rye and wheat breads are superior to white bread in vitamin and protein content or one protein drink.

Mid-morning. When you start to feel tired, grab another piece of fruit for energy. Try a banana, peach, pear, apple, or plum.

Lunch. There are several options for lunch:
Option #1: Baked potato, yam or sweet potato; 4 ounces of nonfat yogurt; and a piece of fruit.
Option #2: 6-8 ounces of non-fat cottage cheese or yogurt; and a piece of fruit.
Option #3: 4-6 ounces of tuna or a chicken breast; 6-8 ounces of pasta or rice; and a piece of fruit.

Mid-afternoon. Piece of fruit.

Dinner. Before your main meal, begin with a huge salad. In addition to being an aid to digestion, it leaves less room in your stomach for the fattening courses that typically follow. But use only low-cal dressing or lemon juice; the fat is in the dressing. And no cold liquid with any meal. It interferes with your digestion. 6-8 ounces of fish or chicken (take off the skin before eating), or veal, lamb, or steak (but remove all visible fat). If you've got a sweet tooth — and most of us do — have a piece of watermelon or some fruit for dessert. Naturally, if you're on a strenuous workout program be sure to increase your snacks during the day for energy. These should include fruits, tuna, pasta, rice, or potatoes.

A FEW MORE GUIDELINES TO BETTER EATING HABITS

• If you must have an occasional steak, trim away the fat. Limit yourself to one or two entrees of meat per week. If you can, dine instead on fish or fowl because red meat will almost always be substantially higher in fat.

• It's not the potato that adds pounds but what the cook does with it. Potatoes sliced and fried in lard or bacon grease are lethal. Sour cream and butter are on my no-no list. Gravy is like drinking fat through a straw. The one and only way to take your potato is baked. If you have to use a topping, add some non-fat sour cream or try a little nonfat ranch dressing.

• For anyone with a sweet tooth, saying farewell to candies, soft drinks, and cookies is a tremendous sacrifice. One answer is honey, the best of all sweeteners, particularly for coffee and tea.

• Milk is important to your diet. It contains calcium and protein; calcium gives you bone density, and protein as you know is essential as well. An early calcium deficiency can increase your chance of osteoporosis later in life. Too much milk, however, may not be good for you, either. If you don't have the proper enzymes to break down milk sugar, it could actually lead to disease. I mix roughly 12 ounces of low-fat milk in my protein drink every morning, and that gives me the calcium I need to help prevent osteoporosis.

• Salt is a killer. It elevates your blood pressure and causes you to retain water. Besides, you get plenty of salt naturally in the foods you eat. And watch out for diet soda. The daughter of a friend once went on a diet and a well disciplined aerobics schedule but couldn't shed a pound. It wasn't until we talked about it that I realized that every day she was drinking 12 to 14 cans of diet drinks which have a lot of sodium.

• Cut down on carbohydrates, I call them White Poisons. Reduce your intake of bread, potatoes, pasta and rice. Whatever you don't metabolize right away will turn into sugar, and sugar turns into fat.

• Stay away from alcohol. It turns into pure sugar.

• Butter is pure fat. It's also loaded with calories. Cooking without butter is both healthier and easier than most people imagine.

• Mayonnaise contains cholesterol-rich egg yolks and is extremely unhealthy.

LEARN HOW TO READ FOOD LABELS

Naturally, we can't subsist on baked potatoes and plain tuna for every meal. The U.S. government's daily dietary guidelines include a healthy meal plan of 3 to 5 servings of vegetables, 2 to 4 servings of fruit, 6 to 11 servings of breads, rice, pasta or grains, and 2 to 3 servings of meat, eggs, poultry, or dried beans, and 2 to 3 servings from the milk, yogurt and cheese group. But a lot of people like to try other foods — like those found in the frozen foods section of your grocery store. The question becomes one of knowledge. Do you know exactly what's in that TV dinner? You've got to learn to read labels because they are crucial tools in your quest for lifelong fitness.

The U.S. government requires that certain foods carry labels with specific facts about nutrition, but "low cholesterol" and "no-fat" claims are often misleading. A "low-fat" label, for example, can mean that a product still derives 45 percent of its total calories from fat. The word "natural" on a label probably refers to its fruit juice content or something similar. It doesn't mean there are no artificial preservatives,and it certainly doesn't mean it's necessarily healthy.

Why is this information important? A certain amount of fat helps fortify the body's immune system, protein builds muscle, and carbohydrates provide energy. Naturally, we need to eat the right proportions of foods in order to give us our daily intake of these nutrients. Food labels also contain information on vitamins and minerals, as well as preservatives and additives.

Be on the lookout for processed foods that contain hidden sugars (dextrose, sucrose, fructose, corn syrup), fat and preservatives. Stay away from products with hydrogenated oils, coconut oil, gums, emulsifiers and especially avoid anything that contains high fructose corn syrup. This is far worse that eating sugar; when it hits your stomach, is absorbed into the blood stream and spikes your insulin level within 10 minutes; then an hour later it plummets, sending your body chemistry into an up and down roller coaster ride.

Try to eat simple, wholesome, unprocessed natural foods (listed below). They're easier to digest and assimilate and don't have adverse side effects. Since it is impossible (and bad for you) to eliminate all fat from your diet, make sure that the fats you do eat are good for you.

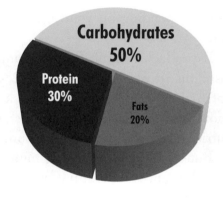

PROTEIN

Salmon
Orange Roughy
Sole
Cod
Tuna
Mackerel
Filet Mignon
Lean Ground Beef (6% fat)
Buffalo
Ostrich
Ground Turkey
Chicken Breast
Chicken Thigh & Legs
Low Fat Cottage Cheese
Low Fat Yogurt
Tofu
Eggs

SIMPLE CARBOHYDRATES

Broccoli
Spinach
Collard Greens
Dark Lettuce
Tomatoes
Red Cabbage
Snap Peas
Peppers
Carrots

COMPLEX CARBOHYDRATES

Yams
Sweet Potatoes
Baked Potatoes
Brown or Wild Rice
Irish Oatmeal
Buckwheat
Barley
Bulgur
Coarse Dark Bread

POLY-UNSATURATED FATS

Flax Seed Oil
Black Currant Oil
Soya Lecithin Oil
Wheat Germ Oil
Light Virgin Olive Oil
Avocados

VITAMINS AND MINERALS

Aging is not a disease, and it's certainly nothing to fear. I'm 80 years old and I'm still as outgoing and productive as I was 30 years ago. I take as much pleasure from life as I can get, and I attribute my good fortune to my dedication to exercise, diet, and the right mental attitude.

Longevity can't be found in any magic pill or medicine. It can't be manufactured in the laboratory. However, there are certain nutrients we can take to help slow down the aging process. If you're getting on in years, you may not be getting enough of these crucial nutrients in your diet. Obviously, a pill can't give you the same range of nutrients as food, but can supplements help?

Most doctors and nutritionists agree that everyone's basic needs can be met by eating a diet rich in vegetables and fruits. But most adults don't even come close. Some of us skip at least one meal a day, while others are on prescription drugs, which can lessen the effectiveness of some nutrients. Depending on your age, you could be suffering from nutrient famine and not even know it.

If you lack vitamin B6, for example, you might suffer from irritability, mental confusion, and insomnia. If you lack vitamin B12, you may be experiencing a lack of energy or some of the signs of Alzheimer's disease. If you lack vitamin C, you could be losing weight or bruising easily. The more you exercise as you get older, the more important is your need for the crucial vitamins and nutrients that maintain strong bones and muscles.

But should you be taking high doses of vitamins to prevent aging? The Recommended Dietary Allowances (RDA) put out by the U.S. government are based on the premise that older Americans need no more vitamins than young adults. But you may need more of certain vitamins and minerals. Why? Because the RDA reflect only those levels that prevent diseases. They don't address what's needed to stay at your peak. Certainly, at the very least, a daily multivitamin/mineral supplement won't hurt anybody.

With a few exceptions, the required amounts of vitamins and minerals for men and women after the age of 50 is the same amount for a 15 year-old. It is also true that as the body ages, it doesn't absorb some nutrients as efficiently as it did when it was younger. Listed in the accompanying table are some of the most common vitamins and nutrients that you may want to incorporate into your diet, along with the RDA, where applicable.

Naturally, none of these supplements should be thought of as a substitute for a sensible, well balanced diet. Moreover, you should never take levels above the RDA without first checking with your doctor. Very high levels of certain vitamins and minerals — iron, for example — can have serious side effects. Take your vitamins with your meal. Be sure to drink plenty of water if you increase your intake of vitamins and minerals. Almost all are water soluble; without the proper water intake they aren't absorbed as readily, defeating the purpose of taking the supplements.

VITAMIN & MINERAL RECOMMENDED DAILY ALLOWANCES

Vitamin A   men: 1,000 micrograms women: 800 micrograms

Vitamin A, along with vitamins C and E — otherwise known as anti-oxidants — appear to be able to neutralize dangerous molecules known as oxygen-free radicals. Free radicals damage your DNA, altering your body's chemistry and killing cells. Scientists believe these free radicals play a major role in the development of cancer, heart and lung disease, and cataracts (the clouding of the lens in the eyes that afflicts 20 percent of Americans over 65). There's also evidence that vitamin A prevents night blindness, viral infections, colds and promotes healthy skin and hair.

Vitamin B6   men: 2 milligrams   women: 1.6 milligrams

Vitamin B6 functions in many of the body's chemical reactions associated with amino acid and protein metabolism. It helps prevent anemia, skin lesions, and nerve damage, and it's also been shown to increase the life expectancies of mice and fruit flies. A lack of vitamin B6 may cause depression and an increased risk of cardiovascular disease.

Vitamin B12   men and women: 2 micrograms

Vitamin B12 helps promote growth by allowing the body to reproduce cells more easily. It also helps release energy in foods and has been known to improve performances in athletes.

Vitamin C   men and women: 60 milligrams

Vitamin C is another potent antioxidant that may actually protect people against heart and lung disease, and cancer. At the very least, it can reduce your levels of free radicals. Unlike many other nutrients, vitamins E and C, and beta carotene (a complex deep orange compound that is naturally abundant in sweet potatoes, carrots, and cantaloupes) are safe to take in amounts higher than the Recommended Dietary Allowance. Vitamin E and C seem also to boost the immune system in healthy older people, raising the possibility that supplements could help thwart life threatening infections. Vitamin C also helps maintain collagen in the skin, healthier blood vessels and beautiful skin.

Vitamin D   men and women: 200 IUs

Vitamin D helps the body absorb calcium and phosphate, which are essential for bone growth and repair. Preliminary evidence from Columbia University and the Harvard Medical School further reveal that vitamin D in combination with parathyroid hormone may actually increase bone density, which would help older people fight the battle against osteoporosis.

Vitamin E   men and women: 10 milligrams

Vitamin E is another antioxidant that may be particularly helpful in preventing free radicals from injuring the heart. A recent study at the University of Toronto showed that supplements of 1,000 IUs a day for 21 days significantly reduced free radical production. Another study at the Human Nutrition Research Center on Aging has shown that supplementing elderly people's diets with vitamin E for one month improves their immune responsiveness. Vitamin E also inhibits the formation of free radicals, and helps the oxygenation of blood, giving you more stamina. It may even have some anti-aging properties.

Since it's hard to get lots of vitamin E from foods, and mounting evidence points to its protective qualities, many scientists now recommend vitamin E supplements for everyone. I do, too.

Vitamin K   men: 80 micrograms   women: 65 micrograms

Vitamin K helps the liver formulate a substance that aids in blood clotting, which prevents bleeding and bruising. It also appears to help bones retain calcium. Loss of calcium is a problem for post-menopausal women. But a recent Dutch study of 1,500 women ages 45 to 80 found that supplements of vitamin K may cut the loss of calcium by half.

Folic Acid   men: 200 micrograms women: 180 micrograms

Folic acid also helps promote growth, probably more so than vitamin B12. It may also help protect against heart disease and nerve damage. According to the Tufts University study, a lack of folic acid may cause neurological changes, such as a drop in alertness and memory ability.

Calcium   men and women: 800 milligrams

Calcium is essential for bone growth and repair. Studies have shown that the body's ability to absorb calcium declines with age. But the Tufts University study demonstrated that weight bearing exercise such as walking and jogging, along with a calcium supplement, helps maintain bone density.

Chromium   men and women: 50-200 micrograms   (estimated as safe and adequate)

Chromium picolinate supplements may help increase the levels of "good" cholesterol (HDL) and decrease the levels of "bad" cholesterol (LDL), according to tests conducted at Bemidjii State University in Minnesota. It also helps regulate blood sugar levels and is important in the metabolism of carbohydrates and fat.

Iron   men and women: 15-20 milligrams

Iron is necessary for the body to form hemoglobin, the compound within red blood cells that transports oxygen. A lack of iron may cause fatigue, irritability, and headaches. But I don't recommend taking iron pills without consulting your doctor.

Magnesium   men: 350 milligrams   women: 280 milligrams

Magnesium is crucial in muscle contractions. Also, sufficient levels of magnesium may help reduce the risk of a number of age related illnesses, including heart disease, stroke, and hypertension.

Selenium   men and women: 2,000 milligrams   (estimated minimum)

Selenium complements vitamin E as an effective anti-oxidant, plays a role in thyroid function, hormone metabolism, supports immune function, reduces free radical production and may protect against cancer and premature aging.

Potassium   men and women: 50 milligrams   (estimated minimum)

Potassium is necessary for healthy nerve and muscle functions. It also has been shown to help reduce high blood pressure, which can help prevent heart disease and death from stroke.

Zinc   men: 15 milligrams   women: 12 milligrams

Zinc helps transport carbon dioxide to the lungs. It also is an essential element for the digestion of proteins. It may even bolster the immune system in some people. Most Americans don't consume enough zinc to meet the RDA recommendations, and since physical activity leads to an increased loss of zinc through sweat, you may want to consider zinc supplements, or increasing your consumption of eggs, seafood, and whole wheat products.

Ginseng

Ginseng is my secret of the Orient. It's what the Chinese athletes claim gave them superhuman strength and endurance during the 1992 Summer Olympics. One study in the Soviet Union demonstrated that daily doses of ginseng increased work endurance in lab animals by 25 percent. It's a medicine tonic made from an ancient recipe that seems to have value as both a tranquilizer and an energy booster. You mix one bag of ginseng with hot water as you would a bag of tea. I drink two cups a day.

MY DAILY INTAKE

A report by the National Research Council warned that supplements in excess of RDA "not only have no known health benefits, but may be detrimental to health." Other experts believe most older Americans don't get adequate nutrition in their diets and need a little help. The choice is yours. Here's a list of my daily intake of vitamins and minerals. You may simply want to focus on changing your eating habits by including in your daily menu more of the foods shown below.

Vitamins	*Food Sources*
Biotin	Peas, beans, oatmeal, milk
Vitamin A (beta carotene)	Milk, dairy products, potatoes, green leafy vegetables, carrots
Vitamin B6	Meats, poultry, fish, fruits, nuts, potatoes
Vitamin B12	Meats, eggs, liver, fish, cereal
Vitamin C	Citrus fruits, raw cabbage, green leafy vegetables
Vitamin D	Fortified milk, egg yolks, salmon
Vitamin E	Nuts, seeds, whole grains
Vitamin K	Leafy vegetables, corn, cereals, dairy products, meats, fruits
Folic acid	Green leafy vegetables, liver

Minerals	*Food Source*
Calcium	Turnips, dairy products, beans, almonds
Chromium	Brewer's yeast, kidneys
Copper	Lobster, oysters, avocados
Iodine	Seafood, seaweed
Iron	Green leafy vegetables, dry beans, whole grains, lean meats
Manganese	Spinach, rice, fruits
Magnesium	Turnips, green vegetables, avocados, whole grains, nuts, fish, bananas
Phosphorus	Grains, milk products, fish, poultry
Potassium	Orange juice, baked potato, bananas, tomatoes, salmon, nuts
Selenium	Grains, wheat germ, seafood, nuts, mushrooms
Zinc	Seafood, wheat, beans, dairy products

FROM RAPTURE TO MADNESS

Once you've changed your eating habits, you may notice that your mood swings are more pronounced. One minute you're energetic and productive, the next minute you're nervous and depressed. Mostly, though, you're hungry. You crave sweets and think of foods you shouldn't be eating. This cycle has to do with how foods affect your blood sugar level.

We all know what it feels like to be tired. If you're tired because you worked too hard or because you trained to fatigue, that's good. But if you're constantly tired, and you don't have the energy to even get out of bed, that's bad. Some doctors call this chronic fatigue. If this sounds like you, it could be there's a problem with your levels of blood sugar or glucose.

Glucose is the basic source of energy for the human body. The amount of glucose in your bloodstream is called your blood sugar level. When this level drops below a specific point, the brain sends a signal to your body demanding more fuel. You know that the quickest fix is refined sugars. Consequently, you reach for a candy bar or a piece of cake. The sugar is converted to glucose and sent back into the bloodstream for immediate energy. What's left is stored and eventually turns to fat. The blood sugar level drops again, and you crave more sweets.

If you had reached for a piece of fruit to satisfy your hunger, the blood sugar level would not have risen so quickly or to as high a level. A steady and consistent flow of glucose would have been slowly released into the bloodstream. This supply would have been sufficient for immediate energy, and you would not have had to experience the "rapture-to-madness syndrome."

All refined sugars (candy, cakes, ice cream, chocolate) cause these drastic fluctuations of your blood sugar level. Maintaining your blood sugar concentration within normal limits is essential to effective dieting and to preserving your health since, the older we get, the more likely we are to develop diabetes.

Eat foods as close to nature as possible to allow your blood sugar levels to remain normal and steady. You need to maintain control of your diet and to make intelligent decisions about eating. In order to keep your wits about you, stay away from the rapture-to-madness syndrome. If you're starting a diet, don't power down a hefty meal the night before, because the next morning your blood sugar level is going to be extremely low and you're going to feel like you need a boost, and another diet will have failed.

If you're over 30 and out of shape, begin your program at a slow pace and be sure to get a preliminary medical examination. As you age, the incidence of certain diseases is higher, particularly heart and lung disease. Nothing is worse than being cut down in the prime of your life by a stroke. Heart disease, especially, is indiscriminate. It strikes both men and women. Most heart attacks or strokes are the result of blocked coronary arteries. These arteries become clogged because of a buildup of cholesterol, a waxy substance that circulates in the bloodstream. So cholesterol is another level you need to keep your eye on.

Cholesterol is a body chemical produced by the liver for a variety of reasons. The one that concerns us is its role in transporting fats in the bloodstream. You can't get along without it, but research has disclosed that you'd better not have too much of it, either. Arteries clogged with cholesterol can become so narrow that blood clots can't pass through. If this happens, blood can't reach the heart, resulting in an attack. But aerobic exercise can eliminate some of these problems; it helps expand the blood vessels and push blood supply to the heart muscle.

A high level of cholesterol is a sure sign of someone who's on the road to cardiovascular disease, especially in the case of older people. Cholesterol clogs the channels through which blood flows. Normally it is purged naturally by the body, but when the cholesterol level is too high, it deposits itself just beneath the walls of the arteries.

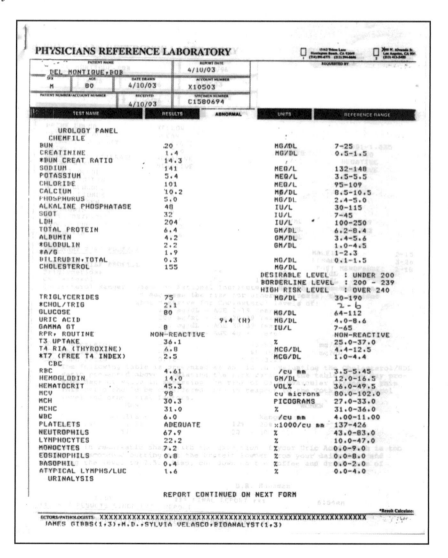

The "normal" cholesterol range is between 150 and 200, but this is misleading because you have to test the "good" cholesterol (high density lipoproteins) against the "bad" cholesterol (low density lipoproteins). It's not enough to simply lower your total cholesterol level. Studies show that even people with healthy cholesterol levels can have dangerously high levels of LDL and dangerously low levels of HDL. I had a friend who kept bragging about his 150 cholesterol level. But when I scrutinized his report, I noticed his HDL was somewhere around the 22 level, but his LDL was off the chart. I looked at him and said, "You're a walking time bomb. Go see a doctor." Fortunately, he took my advice.

If you're watching your cholesterol, the ratio between HDL and LDL should be your primary concern. LDL seems to be responsible for depositing cholesterol in tissue and on the blood vessel walls. HDL seems to do just the opposite — remove cholesterol and carry it back to the liver for disposal. Studies have shown that as the HDL goes up, the rate of heart disease goes down. Women tend to maintain higher HDL levels than men. Exercise also helps raise the blood levels of the "good" cholesterol. The correct combination of HDL and LDL levels gives you your best chance of staving off heart attacks

One of the most deadly causes of increased cholesterol are saturated fats — beef, pork, butter, eggs, lard, and hydrogenated shortening (all trans-fatty acids). You can reduce the amount of cholesterol in your system and decrease your chances of heart disease by eating fish and by using skim and low-fat dairy products. Foods high in fiber may also significantly reduce your blood cholesterol. Some studies suggest that aspirin offers significant protection from strokes by thinning the blood. Aspirin and niacin help keep arteries from clogging up and blocking blood flow to the brain or heart. Check with your physician.

How do you know if you have too much cholesterol in your system? Get your doctor to measure the cholesterol in your blood with a blood lipids test. Of course, you can sometimes get an inaccurate reading. If you find levels that seem way out of whack, be sure to get a second opinion. While you're at it, have your doctor run a complete blood panel test, not just a finger-prick blood test, especially if you're approaching middle age.

I get a blood panel test every six months. It's thorough and complete. I also take a stress test every year. Your body is like a finely tuned machine. You've got to get everything operating at 100 percent efficiency to guarantee your health. Reading the charts from these tests, however, can be like trying to read a foreign language. You'll have the incredible urge to crumple it in your hands and work on your bank shot to the trash can, but don't. Lives have been saved when potential problems were detected early. So here's a rundown (listed alphabetically) of various tests and how they may relate to you (naturally, you'll want to consult your doctor). Keep in mind that these are just the normal ranges, and that some people may easily fall outside these parameters. My tests, like the one pictured below, typically fall within these parameters, with few exceptions.

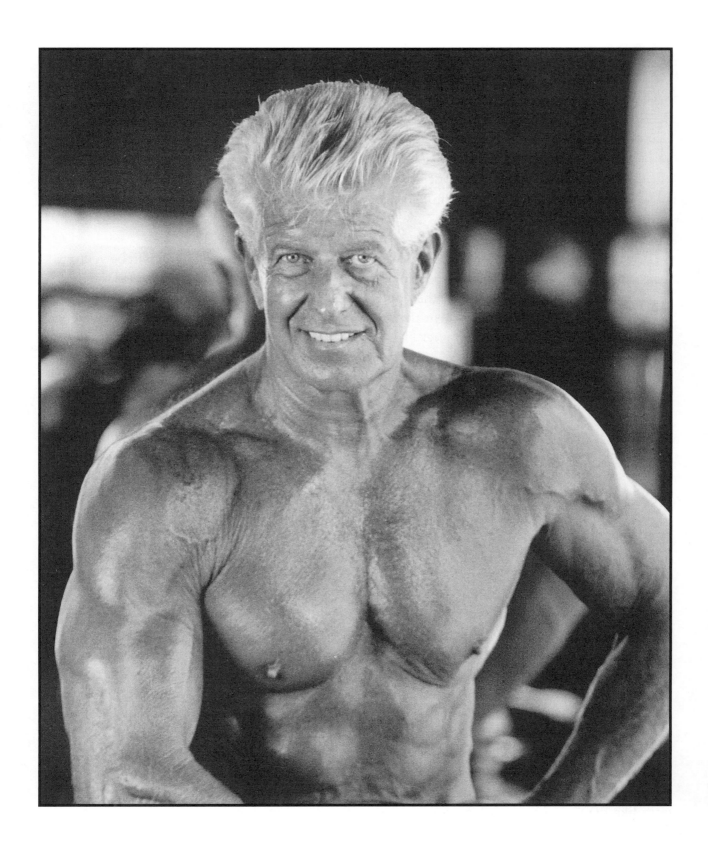

BLOByyy—
BLOOD TESTS

Test	Relates to	Normal Range
Alkaline	Liver/bones	> 17 yrs: 25—140 u/i
Bilirubin (total)	Liver/jaundice	0.2—1.2 mg/dl
Blood Urea Nitrogen	Kidney	7—25 mg/dl
Carbon Dioxide	Fluid balance	22—32 meq/l
Chloride	Fluid balance	96—109 meq/l
Cholesterol (total)	Risk of heart disease/stroke	150—200 mg/dl
HDL	" "	M: 30—75 mg/dl
		F: 40—90 mg/dl
LDL	" "	< 130 mg/dl
Total/HDL Ratio	" "	M: 5.0
		F: 4.4
Creatinine	Kidney	7—25 mg/dl
Ferritin	Iron, anemia	M: 20—450
		F: < 45 yrs: 7—200
		F: > 45 yrs: 10—350
Gamma	Liver	M: 0—65 u/l
		F: 0—45 u/l
Glucose	Pancreas, diabetes	65—115 mg/dl
Glutamyl	Alcoholism	M: 0—65 u/l
		F: 0—45 u/l
Hematocrit	% of red blood cells	M: 4.4—6.2
		F: 3.8—5.4
Hemoglobin	Oxygen, anemia	M: 39%—54%
		F: 35%—48%
Lactic	Liver	100—240 u/l
Phosphatase	Strength	> 17 yrs: 25—140 u/l
Phosphorus	Bones	> 17 yrs: 2.5—4.5mg/dl
Platelet Count	Clotting	140—450
Potassium	Fluid balance	3.5—5.3 meq/l
Protein (total)	Kidney, liver	6.0—8.5 g/dl
Albumin	" "	3.5—5.5 g/dl
Globulin	" "	2.0—3.5 g/dl
Albumin/Globulin Ratio	" "	1.0—2.4
Creatine	Heart muscle	M: 20—220 u/l
		F: 20—150 u/l
Red Blood Count	Anemia	M: 4.4—6.2
		F: 3.8—5.4
SGOT	Liver, hepatitis	0—40 u/l

BLOOD TESTS (continued)

SGPT	Fluid balance	0—45 u/l
Sodium	Fluid balance	135—147 meq/1
Triglycerides	Heart disease	30—150 mg/dl
Uric Acid	Gout	M: 3.0—9.0 mg/dl
		F: 2.2—7.7 mg/dl
White Blood Cell Count	Immune system	4.0—11.0

ARE YOU DRINKING ENOUGH WATER?

Water is almost as necessary to our survival as oxygen. Without it, we can survive only several days. "We even need water to breathe," says Dr. Perry. "Our lungs must be moistened by water to facilitate the intake of oxygen and the excretion of carbon dioxide. We lose approximately a pint of liquid each day just exhaling."

If you're not in "fluid balance," as the medical community calls it, you can actually damage your body's normal functions. Take a look at the consequences of not drinking enough water: a gain in body fat, since water helps with our digestion and metabolism; dehydration, since water helps regulate our body temperature through perspiration; an increase in the toxicity level in your body, because your kidneys need water to filter waste — (this is of particular concern to older people, since the kidney's ability to filter waste slows with age, and inefficient waste removal can be damaging to the kidneys). At the very least, neglecting to compensate for fluid loss, particularly when exercising, can cause lethargy and nausea.

Yet most people haven't a clue as to how much water they should be drinking. In fact, many older people live in a constant state of dehydration — they don't drink enough water because the body's "thirst mechanism" diminishes with age, making dehydration more likely, according to the March 1993 issue of the Johns Hopkins Medical Letter. Water is vital to every aspect of your body's physiological functioning. And the more you exercise, the more water you need to keep your body in fluid balance.

"Water acts as a medium for various chemical reactions in the body," says Dr. Perry. "It carries nutrients and oxygen to the cells through the blood. It helps to regulate our body temperature, and it lubricates our joints. This is particularly important if you're arthritic, have chronic problems with your muscles or bone structure, or are athletically active."

It also helps you maintain good skin and muscle tone, and gives you a beautiful complexion.

So how much water should you drink? Roughly 1/2 ounce per pound of body weight if you're a inactive person (that's 10 8-ounce glasses a day if your weight is 160 pounds), and 2/3 ounce per pound if you're an active person (13 to 14 8-ounce glasses a day). Your water intake should be spread evenly throughout the day, including the evening. And always sip your water, never gulp. You should also always check with your physician before increasing your water intake.

When you first increase your daily water intake you may find yourself running to the bathroom more often. Initially, the bladder will be sensitive to the increased amount of fluid. But after only a few weeks your bladder should calm down. It's important to recognize that there's a difference between water and other beverages, such as diet soda, tea, beer, and fruit juices. Unfortunately, while such drinks contain some water, they also contain substances that are unhealthy. Soda contains sodium. Caffeinated beverages like coffee stimulate the adrenal glands, while fruit juices contain a lot of sugar and stimulate the pancreas.

As for water from the tap or bottled water, I always carry bottled water with me because it's easy to transport. However, at home, I drink water directly from the tap. The bottled water industry is Big Business. Is bottled water any better than tap water? Who really knows? If you can afford bottled water and you like the taste, go for it. If you would prefer to stick to tap water, that's fine, in my opinion. As I said, I do both, depending on which is more convenient.

Proper water intake is an important element in weight loss. If people who are trying to lose weight don't drink enough water, the body can't metabolize the fat. Want to know my secret to good health and longevity? Drink plenty of water and wash all the toxins, impurities, and fats out of your system.

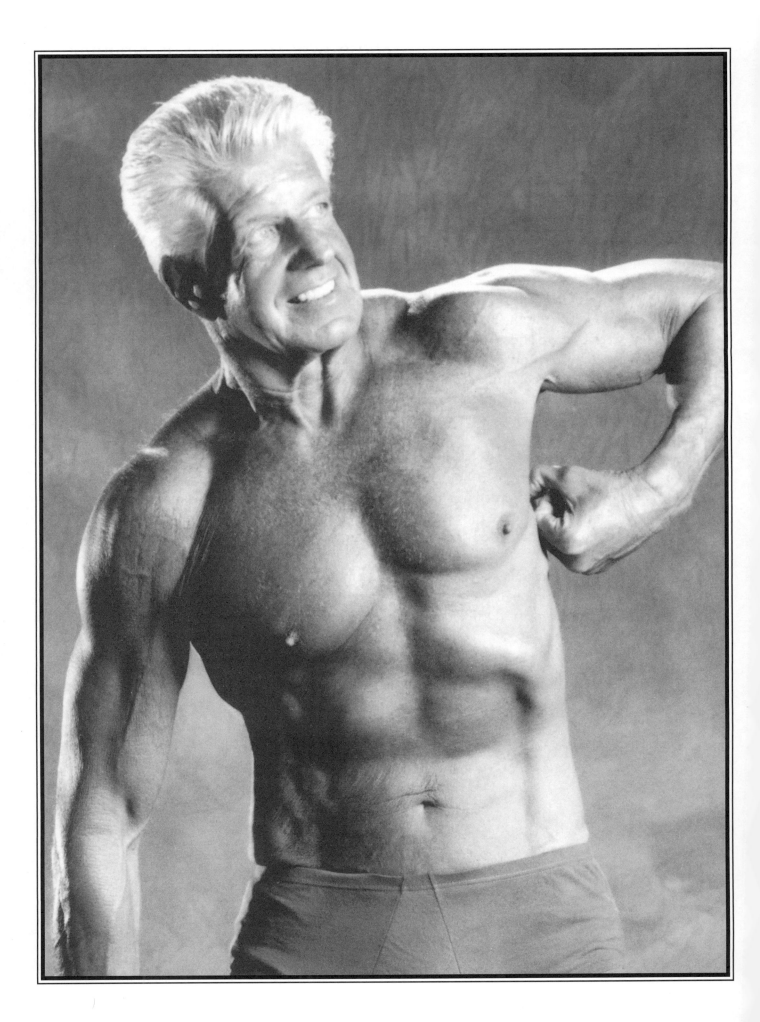

Fine-Tuning Your New Image

Let's be honest, everyone wants to look and feel more attractive. Unfortunately, life often flashes by with no advance warning. You look in the mirror one day and notice, well, certain changes. You may start to see a wrinkle or a few gray hairs. Mostly you'll notice a loss of vigor and strength. But many of these signs can be improved or even corrected with common sense and a few simple exercises. Let's look at some problem areas and their solutions:

STRESS

If you don't think stress plays a significant role in your life, think again. 50 percent of people's health problems are stress related. Do you suffer from an occasional headache, neck or back pain, or high blood pressure? Strong emotions release adrenaline and other stress-related chemicals into the blood stream. Medical science's best guess is that these chemicals play a significant role in most or even all of the long-term chronic illnesses including heart disease, kidney and liver failure, maybe even cancer.

One of the best ways to reduce the stress in your life is through a sensible exercise program and regular meditation. Here are a few uncomplicated suggestions to rid yourself of those tension filled aches and pains:

- Whenever you feel tense, do a few push-ups, sit-ups, knee bends, or take a few deep breaths — anything that will take your mind off your troubles.
- Assign yourself without guilt to some form of recreation — golf, fishing, tennis, hiking, or even biking. Such a pastime is not a luxury but a prescribed necessity if you wish to stay healthy.
- Learn to breathe correctly. Proper breathing supplies oxygen to the blood, slows down respiration, and triggers the body's relaxation response.
- Eat a balanced diet. Poor eating habits can deprive you of vitamins and minerals needed for good health. Check into anti-stress vitamins and minerals.
- Cut back on your intake of caffeine, which tends to make people nervous and tense. Drink ginseng instead.
- Take a brisk walk. It often does more good for an unhappy but otherwise healthy adult than all the medicine and psychology in the world.
- Try meditation. Add yoga to your daily exercise routine.
- Take a hot bath with lavender oil.

POSTURE

A correct posture also helps control stress, but it has many other benefits as well. Gravity is constantly pulling down anything we don't hold up. As we age, the neck begins to move forward, causing the back to slouch. To compensate, one must improve the "postural muscles" that, when fatigued and weakened allow our bodies to sag and slump. Obviously, the more you slump, the more you lose flexibility, so you not only look older, you move older and feel older — which causes more back problems, and even more stress. That's why posture and balance are prerequisites to a naturally healthy body.

Start by walking tall, with your pubic bone tucked up and into your navel, and your stomach muscles tight. The person who carries him or herself with dignity and pride is more likely to come across as attractive and desirable. Good posture means good balance. Your weight should be evenly distributed from your heels to the balls of your feet and toes. Your center of gravity should be slightly in front of and between your ankles. If we were to draw an imaginary line, it would run upward from that point through the midpoint between your knees, your pubic bone, your navel, the midpoint of your sternum, the mid-tip of your chin, between your eyes, and straight up through your forehead.

The arches of your feet should be relaxed and slightly raised on the inside. Your ankles should be at the same level horizontally, and so should your knees hips, shoulders, eyes, and ears. Your arms should hang relaxed, and your hands and fingertips should be level. Ask yourself a few basic questions: Do I stand too much on my heels? Are my feet too flat, with no arches evident? Do I lock my knees? Do I stick my buttocks out and give myself a swayed lower back? Do I round my shoulders so much that my head is sticking out and I look like a turkey? It took me years to understand how to keep my body coordinated and balanced. Since then, I've used a technique taught by Dr. Perry for maintaining correct posture.

Imagine yourself with five helium-filled balloons tied to your body — one red balloon attached to the top of your head, two white balloons to each pectoral muscle, and two blue balloons to the top of each hip bone. Visualize the balloons lifting gently, but firmly, your head, chest, and hips. It's as if you're stretching the knots out of your spinal cord. This alignment is close to perfect. If it doesn't come naturally, practice. In a few weeks, you should feel more graceful, more confident, even younger. When you walk, pretend that you are 7 feet tall.

GROOMING HABITS

Less serious, but no less important to your overall image, are the little things in life — namely, grooming habits. Men tend to lose hair where they want it and grow hair where they don't. A woman's hair tends to thin and to lose some of its youthful sheen. The only way to maintain the health of hair is to prevent damage, which can be caused by everyday occurrences — ultraviolet radiation from the sun, harsh chemicals, excess heat from a hair dryer. Pay attention to the details. What's the point of prolonging your life through exercise and diet if you can't take care of the more unsightly aspects of aging?

Your skin, for example, reveals the outer you. If you want to feel younger, you've got to maintain younger looking skin and that means a life free of stress and fatigue. Here are some other suggestions:

• Stick to an exercise program. It will help replenish elastic fibers in the skin while sweating promotes an increased flow of nutrients to the skin and enhances the removal of impurities.

• Maintain a low-fat diet. Be sure to take your vitamins, especially B complex vitamins, and vitamins A and C (found in fresh fruits and vegetables). Ingesting flaxseed and black currant oils also tends to improve the overall look of your skin.

• Don't smoke. Smoking is not only bad for your health, but it's bad for your skin. It tends to decrease blood supply to the small blood vessels under the skin, which can exacerbate wrinkling

• Avoid overindulging in alcohol. You tend to "puff up" in the morning after too much drink, and that temporarily stretches the skin, causing wrinkles to form. It also tends to rupture the tiny capillaries in your face.

• Avoid stress. It causes worry lines.

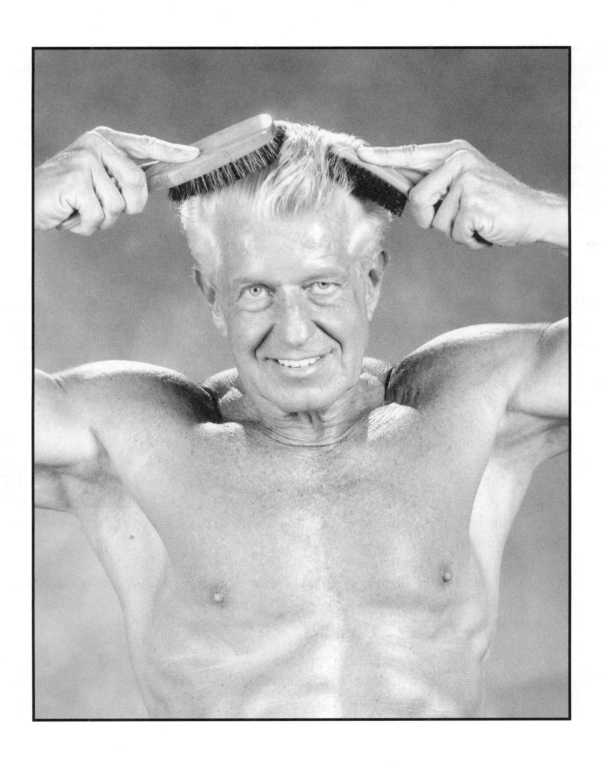

You may know some people who seem to have naturally old looking skin. More than likely it's the result of a diet high in fats, especially if that person spends a lot of time outdoors. Sunlight tends to turn fats into tissue damaging molecules. It can, in fact, accelerate aging of the skin when the tissues are deficient in protective vitamins and natural substances, according to Dr. Zane Kime, one of the world's foremost authorities on sunlight and health. Too much sun can cause burns, premature aging, and skin cancer, which is why a lot of doctors advise against sunbathing. And I'm not about to recommend overexposing your body to the harmful rays. But I've learned from personal experience that a certain amount of sunlight can actually improve your overall health. Have you ever noticed, for example, how a sunny day seems to revive your spirits? Dr. Kime claims sunlight can lower high blood pressure, decrease cholesterol, and increase resistance to certain diseases. I've found that it enhances the beauty of my skin. A tan body just looks healthier to me than a pale one.

Finally, chances are good that you already brush and floss twice a day. And I'm sure you get your teeth cleaned twice a year by a professional. But have you started noticing stains on your teeth that you can't erase? The problem is not your age, but rather bacteria living in your mouth that dissolve tooth enamel and infect the gums. Maintaining healthy teeth is not that difficult. All it really takes is common sense. Eat a healthy diet, stay away from sugars and sweets, and watch out for coffee stains. Most of these problems can be corrected either through proper cleaning or by consulting your dentist.

SEX

Everything I've outlined here should help you feel more attractive and more energized. Which brings me to the issue of sex. Just as important as keeping fit is your ability to continue to have sex. Giving up on this pastime at any age will drain not only your self-confidence but also the vitality from your marriage, your work, even the second half of your life. In recent years, scientists have discovered that changes in sexual function occur as we get older. Testosterone levels in men drop after the age of 40. Women, of course, experience menopause. These hormone deficiencies can cause low sexual desire.

If the sexual tides are beginning to ebb, it could be that you're too weak and tired to think about sex, or that you lack strength in key muscular areas. It doesn't take bulging biceps and four-minute-mile stamina to have a successful love life. But our bodies are like finely tuned machines. Certainly if you're not at your best physically you're not at your best sexually. Even your diet could affect your sexual prowess. Too much fat, for example, tends to slow down your metabolism and cause a build-up of plaque inside blood vessels that are crucial to your performance in the bedroom.

Research indicates, however, that improved muscular response, endurance, and cardiovascular/respiratory capacity almost guarantee better sexual encounters and greater sexual enjoyment. In other words, exercise can improve and stimulate the body's sexual response by improving the circulation to organs and bodily regions.

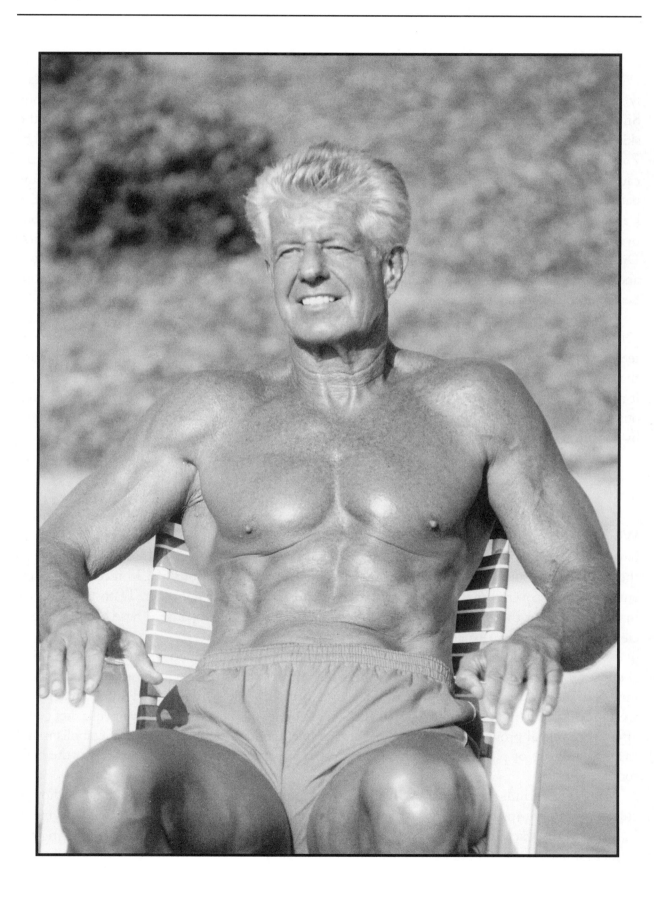

One of the most exciting developments I've discovered in the research on hormones and aging is that you've got the ability to build your confidence and improve your love life through physical conditioning. Whether you're 40 and suffer from low self-esteem, or 60 and suffering from physical changes associated with aging, you don't have to be deprived of sexual enjoyment. Working out can lead to better cardiovascular response and better blood flow. Furthermore, sex requires a certain amount of stamina and muscle movements. Doesn't it make sense, then, that a physically fit person is guaranteed better sexual encounters and greater sexual enjoyment? So what's the link between exercise and sex?

- When your body's in shape, you feel more attractive and others are more attracted to you.
- Some studies show that exercise promotes testosterone and estrogen release, increases blood flow to the sexual organs and activates your libido.
- Exercise improves heart and lung functions, which keep people healthy enough to enjoy sex as they get older.
- Psychologically, people who exercise feel better about themselves, and have a healthier attitude about their sexual relationships.
- Gives you more energy and more stamina.

Understanding the changes that come about as a result of aging is the first step to dealing with problems in the bedroom or elsewhere. Ultimately, though, it will be up to each aging person to decide how he or she wants to fiddle with destiny. Maintain your proper weight, keep up your health, and eat a low-fat diet, and you'll be on the road to a longer, healthier life. As long as you continue to push yourself physically, and take care of yourself mentally and emotionally, you've got a much better chance of maintaining vigor, strength, and endurance.

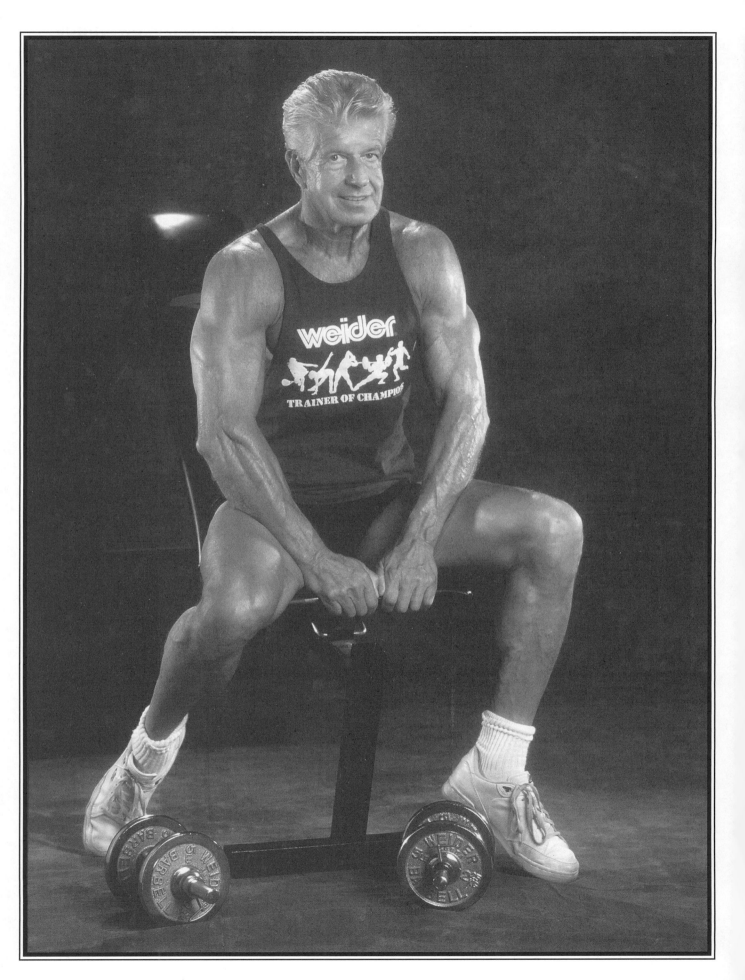

Achieving Lifelong Fitness

Even today, there are scientists who believe your life is controlled by an inner body clock that sets the time for aging and death. Whether you will live to be 63 or 93 is hard to predict. Although it's true that a strong gene pool plays a factor in the overall equation, I believe each one of us has the capacity to live 100 years or more. It's only through the abuses of modern society and unhealthy life-styles that we've managed to terminate our lives so early.

Aging is not based on the number of years you've lived, but on how you've lived your years, and mistakes made when we're younger can have serious repercussions later in life. When exactly do you reach middle age? How old is old? People who live to see their sixtieth birthday without acquiring heart disease, diabetes, or some other illness stand a good chance of living at least another quarter of a century. Many of the problems we typically associate with old age-weak muscles and a poor cardiovascular system, diabetes, memory loss, and a waning interest in sex — can be prevented with a regular exercise program and a proper diet.

Trying to slow down the clock of aging, however, is not so much a straight line as a series of advances and retreats. You might cheat on your diet or skip a workout. Everyone does. But the more you believe that strength training, diet, and cardiovascular conditioning are the most important components of good health, the less you have to worry about an inner body clock. Activity is life, stagnation is death — and lack of physical activity is just plain stupid.

But you've got to keep at it because the benefits of exercise are short lived. Once you stop, within a short time your blood-sugar tolerance returns to pretraining levels, and the gains you've made from lifting weights, running, and eating well start to reverse themselves In fact when conditioned people stop training they lose what they've gained at a much faster rate than they gained it. Undoubtedly, the toughest hurdle to a better, healthier life is motivation. The older you get, the tougher it is to get going. Working out in a gym in front of the young guns of the world may not sound like the best way to build your self-esteem. On the other hand, it may be just what you need to rejuvenate your spirits. You've got to have a good positive mental attitude, because you are as you think. A lot of people say, "I'm going to do it," but fail at even trying. You've got to be more specific. You've got to have goals. You've got to have a mental image of what you want to look like and who you want to be. And you've got to have commitment. It will take you a while to get into the habit of exercise. Psychologists say it takes 21 days to establish a pattern and 100 days (about 14 weeks) to make it automatic. If you can get past those first three months, you stand an extremely good chance of staying committed to a goal of lifelong fitness.

It's about taking charge of your life by tapping your inner resources. Make the small changes first. Start by walking or changing your diet. Small changes lead to bigger changes. Good habits are the keys to success, while poor habits will get you nowhere.

Our society has a tendency to attach stigmas to its middle-aged and older members. We're supposed to look forward to retirement, but it's this kind of attitude that makes us, well, old. The more you sit around complaining about feeling old, about whether age is creeping up on you, the faster your body will give out on you.

Stay busy and involved. If you're like me, you may have found that the busier you are, the happier you are — and the more you take on, the more you get done. It seems to me that during the periods when I'm at my most active, I never get sick — it just doesn't occur to me, and even if it did, I couldn't afford the time. The energy and attention I get from working out, along with the good health, are the three primary factors that motivate me to continue. People don't come up to me and say I look great — for an old man. They come up to me and say I look great — for any man.

I've identified seven workable and proven secrets of longevity. These are simple and practical personal improvement tips for those of you who want the best from life.

THE SEVEN DOORS TO GOOD HEALTH

Exercise • Diet • Rest • Fresh air • Sunshine • Water • Mental attitude

It has been observed that those who exercise live longer than those who don't, and that loss of muscle mass and strength is the result, not of the normal aging process, but of an ever increasing sedentary life-style. You cannot reduce fat, build muscle, and live longer under your own terms unless you've got the proper nutrients and exercise programs, and the proper mental attitude. Your health is your wealth. You can grow old gracefully, or stay young gracefully. The decision ultimately is yours.

THE SEVEN SPIRITUAL LAWS

1) Good habits are the key to success, poor habits unlock the door to failure.

2) I shall greet the day with love in my heart; I shall have love for myself, I shall have pride, I shall have self-esteem and I shall have self-respect because you cannot give what you don't have. This is the most important ingredient.

3) I shall persist until I succeed. If I fail, I shall try and try again, I shall persist until I succeed because I am nature's greatest miracle and nature knows not defeat. She eventually emerges victorious.

4) I shall live this day as if it is my last, yesterday is gone and tomorrow may never come. I shall act today with conviction because most people put off until tomorrow and tomorrow may never come.

5) I shall be emotionally stable, I shall be consistent and I shall be happy.

6) I shall laugh and smile and be happy because happy people like happy people and I also get my positive juices flowing through my body to make things happen.

7) I shall have a burning desire which is nothing but a mental image of what one day will be – then I will have faith, belief, enthusiasm and hope, because I believe with faith, belief, enthusiasm and hope you can accomplish what ever you want to accomplish.

I believe you can do anything you want to do. Be whatever you want to be. And go wherever you want to go. Provided you want it enough, there is nothing you cannot accomplish in life if you want it bad enough.

Index

Bob Delmonteque's Shopping List

Youth Cocktail
www.asseenonamericantv.com/youth_cocktail.htm

Gero Vita International
www.gvi.com

Weider Nutrition
www.weider.com

Standard Process Labs
Phone 800-372-7218
Fax 800-431-7662

Doctor Green's First
www.greenfirst.com

Whole Foods
www.wholefoodsmarket.com

Young Living Essential Oils
Phone 801-418-8900
Fax 801-418-8888

Hormone RX
www.mypainmeds.com

Dr. Tony Quinn's Mind Master Program
www.tonyquinn.com

Dr. Young, Inner Light
www.innerlight.com

Genrich Pharmacy
email: sjpharm@aol.com

Kronus Labs
Phone 602-667-5623

Power Plate
www.power-plate.com

Bibliography

Books

Abernethy, Jean Beaven. Old Is Not a Four—Letter Word! New York Abingdon Press, 1975.

American Physical Fitness Research Institute. Here's to Wellness. New York: Vanguard Press, 1984.

Anderson, Bob. Stretching. Bolinas, CA: Shelter Publications, 1980.

Brooks, Marvin B. Lifelong Sexual Vigor. New York: Doubleday, 1981.

Cooper, Kenneth H. Aerobics. New York: Bantam Books, 1968.

Diamond, Harvey and Marilyn. Fit for Life. New York: Warner Books, 1985.

Douglas, Ben H. AgeLess. Mississippi: Quail Ridge Press, 1990.

Evans, William, and Irwin H. Rosenberg. Biomarkers: The 10 Determinants of Aging You Can Control New York: Simon & Schuster, 1991.

Fixx, Jim. Jim Fixx's Second Book of Running. New York: Random House, 1980.

FutureYouth. Pennsylvania: Rodale Press, 1987.

Glass, Justine C. Live to Be 180. New York: Taplinger, 1961.

Haas, Robert. Eat to Win. New York: Rawson Associates, 1983.

Keeton, Kathy. Longevity. New York: Penguin, 1992.

LaLanne, Jack. The Jack LaLanne Way to Vibrant Good Health. Englewood Cliffs, NJ: Prentice-Hall, Inc., 1960.

McLish, Rachel, with Bill Reynolds. Flex Appeal. New York: Warner Books, 1984.

Parker, Robert B., and John R. Marsh. Training with Weights. New York: J. B. Lippincott Peale, Norman Vincent. The Power of Positive Thinking New York: Prentice—Hall, Inc., 1952.

Samuels, Mike, and Nancy Samuels. The Well Adult. New York: Summit Books, 1988.

Simons, Harvey B., and Steven R. Levisohn. The Athlete Within: A Personal Guide to Total Fitness. Boston: Little, Brown, 1987.

Newspaper Articles

Condon, Garret. "Stretch Those Muscles: It's a New Way to Stay Healthy." Los Angeles Times, July 17, 1992, p. E9.

Doheny, Kathleen. "Pump Iron to Reverse Effects of Age." Los Angeles Times, July 4, 1992, p. E6.

Hanc, John. "Ten Great Myths of Physical Fitness." Newsday, November 10, 1985.

Magazine Articles

Deters, Tom. "Training Past 40." Muscle & Fitness, August 1991, p. 129.

Epstein, Randi Hutter. "Do Men Go Through Menopause?" M Magazine, July 1992, p. 31.

Hepburn, Katharine. "No Excuses? Keep on Trying!" TV Guide, October 19, 1985, p. 12.

Keeton, Kathy. "Mental Muscle." Omni, May 1992, p. 40.

Laliberte, Richard. "Stay Younger Longer." Men's Health, June 1992, p. 46.

Prokop, Dave. "New Approaches to Beating Back Pain." Muscle & Fitness, November 1991, p. 118.

Roark, Anne C. "Fitness Past 40." Los Angeles Times Magazine, October 8, 1989, p. 46.

Stocker, Sharon. "How Great Can a Person Look at 50—Plus?" Prevention, October 1991, p. 77.

Strock, Richard. "The New Case for Resistance Training." Club Business International, May 1992, p. 26.

Toufexis, Anastasia. "The New Scoop on Vitamins." Time, April 6, 1992, p. 54.

University of California at Berkeley Wellness Letter. "Nutrition and Exercise: What Your Body Needs." Volume 9, Issue 8, May 1993, pp. 4-6.

Weider, Joe. "The Weider Body—Building Lifestyle." Muscle & Fitness, May 1992, p. 98.

Weider, Joe. "85 and Going Strong: How Bodybuilding Keeps You Youthful and Strong for Truly Vital Golden Years." Muscle & Fitness, March 1992, p. 158.

INDEX

INDEX